Current Status of Carotid
Bifurcation Angioplasty
and Stenting

Current Status of Carotid Bifurcation Angioplasty and Stenting

edited by

Frank J. Veith

Montefiore Medical Center–Albert Einstein College of Medicine
New York, New York

Max Amor

U.C.C.I. Polyclinique d'Essey
Essey-les-Nancy, France

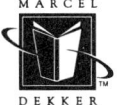

MARCEL DEKKER, INC.   NEW YORK · BASEL

ISBN: 0-8247-0495-9

This book is printed on acid-free paper.

Headquarters
Marcel Dekker, Inc.
270 Madison Avenue, New York, NY 10016
tel: 212-696-9000; fax: 212-685-4540

Eastern Hemisphere Distribution
Marcel Dekker AG
Hutgasse 4, Postfach 812, CH-4001 Basel, Switzerland
tel: 41-61-261-8482; fax: 41-61-261-8896

World Wide Web
http://www.dekker.com

The publisher offers discounts on this book when ordered in bulk quanti-ties. For more information, write to Special Sales/Professional Market-ing at the headquarters address above.

Current printing (last digit):
10 9 8 7 6 5 4 3 2 1

PRINTED IN THE UNITED STATES OF AMERICA

Preface

New endovascular treatments have generated much controversy. The inherently less invasive nature of these treatments renders them attractive to physicians and patients alike. Often these new modalities for treating vascular lesions are widely embraced and their use vigorously advocated before appropriate evaluations of safety, efficacy, and effectiveness have been documented. Moreover, different specialties may deem themselves better equipped to administer these new treatments than the specialties that utilize more traditional treatment modalities. This generates further conflict, controversy, claims, and counterclaims. Both the medical profession at large and patients may be left confused and ill-served by all this polarization.

We postulated that a series of consensus conferences, appropriately structured and documented, might help to dispel this confusion and provide the medical profession at large with points of agreement, a solid base of information, and unified or prevailing informed opinions that can guide physicians in advising patients regarding the appropriate role of the new endovascular treatment.

Certainly carotid bifurcation angioplasty and stenting for arteriosclerotic stenotic lesions represents a relatively new endovascular treatment that is highly controversial. It seemed most appropriate to us that we begin our consensus conference approach to new endovascular treatments by addressing this topic.

Frank J. Veith
Max Amor

Contents

Contributors

Nadim Al-Mubarak, M.D.   Department of Interventional Cardiology, Lenox Hill Heart and Vascular Institute of New York, New York, New York

Max Amor, M.D.   Codirector, Cardiovascular Unit, Department of Cardiology, U.C.C.I. Polyclinique d'Essey, Essey-les-Nancy, France

Hugh G. Beebe, M.D.   Clinical Professor, Department of Surgery, University of Michigan Medical School, Ann Arbor, Michigan, and Director, Jobst Vascular Center, Toledo, Ohio

Peter R. F. Bell, M.D., F.R.C.S.   Professor, Department of Surgery, University of Leicester, and University Hospitals of Leicester NHS Trust, Leicester Royal Infirmary, Leicester, England

Patrice Frank Bergeron, M.D. Chief, Department of Thoracic and Cardiovascular Surgery, Foundation Hospital Saint Joseph, Marseilles, France

Amman Bolia, M.B.Ch.B., D.M.R.D., F.R.C.R. Consultant Interventional Vascular Radiologist, Department of Radiology, University Hospitals of Leicester NHS Trust, Leicester Royal Infirmary, Leicester, England

J. J. Connors III, M.D. Director, Interventional Neuroradiology, Radiology Services, Inova Fairfax Hospital, Falls Church, Virginia

Edward B. Diethrich, M.D. Medical Director, Arizona Heart Institute and Arizona Heart Hospital, Phoenix, Arizona

Gustav R. Eles, D.O., F.A.C.C. Department of Cardiology, Pittsburgh Vascular Institute, University of Pittsburgh Medical Center–Shadyside Hospital, Pittsburgh, Pennsylvania

Richard D. Fessler, M.D. Assistant Clinical Professor and Director of Neurovascular Surgery, Department of Neurosurgery, Wayne State University, Detroit, Michigan

Lee R. Guterman, M.D., Ph.D. Assistant Professor, Department of Neurosurgery and Toshiba Stroke Research Center, State University of New York at Buffalo, Buffalo, New York

Isabelle Henry, M.D. Cardiovascular Unit, Department of Cardiology, U.C.C.I. Polyclinique d'Essey, Essey-les-Nancy, France

Michel Henry, M.D. Cardiovascular Unit, Department of Cardiology, U.C.C.I. Polyclinique d'Essey, Essey-les-Nancy, France

Robert W. Hobson II, M.D.　Professor and Director, Division of Vascular Surgery, University of Medicine and Dentistry of New Jersey–New Jersey Medical School, Newark, New Jersey

L. Nelson Hopkins, M.D.　Professor and Chairman, Department of Neurosurgery and Toshiba Stroke Research Center, State University of New York at Buffalo, Buffalo, New York

Michèle Hugel, R.N.　Cardiovascular Intervention Unit, Department of Cardiology, U.C.C.I. Polyclinique d'Essey, Essey-les-Nancy, France

Sriram S. Iyer, M.D.　Interventional Cardiologist and Director of Peripheral Interventions, Lenox Hill Heart and Vascular Institute of New York, New York, New York

Chester R. Jarmolowski, M.D.　Director, Pittsburgh Vascular Institute, and Department of Diagnostic Imaging, University of Pittsburgh Medical Center–Shadyside Hospital, Pittsburgh, Pennsylvania

Barry T. Katzen, M.D., F.A.C.C., F.S.C.V.I.R.　Medical Director, Miami Cardiac and Vascular Institute, Miami, Florida

Patrick G. Khanoyan, M.D.　Cardiologist, Department of Thoracic and Cardiovascular Surgery, Foundation Hospital Saint Joseph, Marseilles, France

Christos Klonaris, M.D.　Vascular Surgeon, Department of Cardiology, U.C.C.I. Polyclinique d'Essey, Essey-les-Nancy, France

Gishel New, M.B., B.S., Ph.D.　Director, Clinical Research, Cardiovascular Research Foundation, Department of Interventional Cardiology, Lenox Hill Heart and Vascular Institute of New York, New York, New York

Takao Ohki, M.D. Chief of Endovascular Programs, Division of Vascular Surgery, Montefiore Medical Center–Albert Einstein College of Medicine, New York, New York

Paul André Pietri, M.D. Department of Thoracic and Cardiovascular Surgery, Foundation Hospital Saint Joseph, Marseilles, France

Vincent Maurice Louis Piret, M.D. Department of Thoracic and Cardiovascular Surgery, Foundation Hospital Saint Joseph, Marseilles, France

Adnan I. Qureshi, M.D. Assistant Professor, Department of Neurosurgery and Toshiba Stroke Research Center, State University of New York at Buffalo, Buffalo, New York

Andrew J. Ringer, M.D. Endovascular Fellow, Department of Neurosurgery and Toshiba Stroke Research Center, State University of New York at Buffalo, Buffalo, New York

Gary S. Roubin, M.D., Ph.D., F.R.A.C.P., F.A.C.C. Chief, Endovascular Section, Department of Interventional Cardiology, Lenox Hill Heart and Vascular Institute of New York, New York, New York

Walter A. Tan, M.D., M.S. Director of Clinical Research and Staff Interventionalist, Departments of Cardiology and Radiology, Pittsburgh Vascular Institute, University of Pittsburgh Medical Center–Shadyside Hospital, Pittsburgh, Pennsylvania

Frank J. Veith, M.D., F.A.C.S. Professor and Chief, Vascular Surgical Services, and Vice Chairman, Department of Surgery, Montefiore Medical Center–Albert Einstein College of Medicine, New York, New York

Jiri J. Vitek, M.D., Ph.D. Department of Interventional Cardiology, Lenox Hill Heart and Vascular Institute of New York, New York, New York

Mark H. Wholey, M.D. Chairman, Pittsburgh Vascular Institute, University of Pittsburgh Medical Center–Shadyside Hospital, Pittsburgh, Pennsylvania

Michael H. Wholey, M.D., M.B.A. Chief, Cardiovascular and Interventional Radiology, University of Texas Health Science Center at San Antonio, San Antonio, Texas

James Robert Wilentz, M.D. Assistant Professor, Department of Medicine, Albert Einstein College of Medicine–Beth Israel Medical Center, New York, New York

Jay S. Yadav, M.D. Department of Cardiology, The Cleveland Clinic Foundation, Cleveland, Ohio

1
Introduction

Frank J. Veith
Montefiore Medical Center–Albert Einstein College of Medicine, New York, New York

Max Amor
U.C.C.I. Polyclinique d'Essey, Essey-les-Nancy, France

I. BACKGROUND AND PURPOSE OF THE CONSENSUS CONFERENCE AND DOCUMENTATION

Balloon angioplasty has been used sporadically for many years to treat carotid bifurcation stenoses (1,2). However, it was only after intravascular stents became available that any enthusiasm was generated for the endovascular treatment of these lesions (3–6). Despite the fact that angiographically favorable results were often achieved, the procedural stroke rates in many of the earlier series remained higher than those for carotid endarterectomy (5–7). Nevertheless, with better selection of patients and improved technology, lower periprocedural stroke rates were observed with carotid bifurcation angioplasty and stenting (CBAS) (8,9). As a result, some workers have proclaimed that CBAS is currently equivalent to or superior to carotid endarterectomy and that CBAS should be widely practiced and used to treat carotid stenoses. This has led to much controversy and equally strong recommendations by others that CBAS not be used widely and that recommendations to do so are inappropriate and unethical at this time (7,10,11). In most of the conflicting reports on this topic, there is far more emotion than data, far more heat than light. The result is that the medical profession at large is left confused by the conflicting claims and recommendations of the overenthusiastic supporters or rabid detractors of CBAS. Accordingly, they have difficulty in determining what treatment is best for their patients and they cannot provide them with rational recommendations.

The purposes of applying the consensus process to CBAS are 1) to assemble the experts in this area, 2) to examine their opinions regarding this method of treatment, and 3) to reach agreement (consensus or near consensus) on what is known, what is not known (disagreement), and what new information is needed. This consensus process is intended to thereby provide a rational overview of CBAS.

In this way the medical community at large can gain a balanced understanding of this new treatment and where it should currently and appropriately be applied in the treatment of patients with carotid bifurcation stenoses due to arteriosclerosis.

II. STRUCTURE OF THE CONSENSUS CONFERENCE AND DOCUMENTATION

To provide the best overview of the topic, the consensus conference organizers, Frank Veith and Max Amor, selected as participants those individuals who were generally acknowledged to be the best and brightest leaders in the field. This meant those physicians who, irrespective of the specialty they represented, had the widest experience and greatest interest in CBAS. Seventeen participants were chosen from four different specialties (interventional radiology, interventional cardiology, vascular surgery, and neurosurgery) and four different countries (United States, United Kingdom, Germany, and France). As shown in Table 1,

Table 1 Participants

Radiologists	Cardiologists	Surgeons
Bolia[a]	Henry[a]	Beebe
Connors[a]	Roubin[a]	(Bell)
Ferguson[a]	Yadav[a]	Bergeron[a]
(Katzen)[a]		Diethrich[a]
(Matthias)[a]		Hobson
(Theron)[a]		Hopkins[a,b]
(Wholey)[a]		Ohki[a]

[a] Major endovascular therapist.
[b] Neurosurgeon.
Participants in parentheses contributed to the questionnaire but were unable to attend the oral session.

seven of these participants were interventional radiologists, three were interventional cardiologists, and seven were surgeons (six vascular surgeons and one neurosurgeon). All 17 participants had a clear endovascular orientation, and all but three were major endovascular therapists. Thus the conference participants were unlikely to represent the views of "surgical foxes guarding the carotid stenosis henhouse" as one participant had worried about when the conference was in the planning stage. All conference participants had evinced an interest in CBAS, had performed clinical or laboratory studies in this field, and had published and lectured widely on this topic. All 17 of the selected participants agreed to take part in the consensus process.

A. Before the Oral Consensus Conference

All 17 participants were sent a questionnaire requesting their responses to 15 key questions relating to the present status of CBAS. These questions were designed to evaluate current points of agreement or disagreement about the present role of CBAS in medical practice. The answers to these questions plus discussion of these questions and their answers at the oral consensus session would serve as a major basis for the consensus document that would result from the consensus process. The questionnaire had room for comments in addition to the "yes," "no," or "uncertain" answers that were possible for most of the questions.

All 17 participants returned their completed questionnaire in time for the answers to be collated and analyzed before the oral session. Thus, the answers to the questions could be discussed effectively at the oral session.

All 17 participants agreed also to contribute a chapter to be included in the book that would serve as the primary documentation of the consensus process. These chapters could express each participant's opinions or predictions about CBAS. They could also include a summary of each author's experience and other views or attitudes about the topic.

In addition, one of the participants felt that an additional three questions should be asked, answered, and discussed at the oral session so that a better, more complete overview of CBAS might be obtained. These three questions were also circulated and answered by all 17 participants. Analysis of these three additional questions was also completed so that they could be discussed at the oral session.

B. Oral Consensus Session

This session was held in New York City on November 21, 1999. Twelve participants in addition to Frank Veith and Max Amor attended. Five participants were unable to attend because of prior commitments or urgent conflicts. One absent participant's views were represented at the oral session by his colleague who was in attendance (Amman Bolia for Peter Bell). Questions and comments from an audience of 250 interested physicians were also entertained by the oral session participants.

The oral session consisted of a 10-min introductory statement outlining the *purpose and structure* of the oral session and the planned documentation that would result. A *summary and analysis* of the answers to each of the 18 questions asked in the questionnaires was then presented. *Discussion of each question and its answers* then followed. In some cases questions were modified to permit answers that most participants could agree to. In other instances participants' answers were changed as the question was clarified by the discussion. An effort was made by all to reach consensus or near consensus on as many aspects of CBAS as was currently possible.

Following these discussions of each question, each of the 12 participants in attendance presented a 5–10-min *oral summary* of the key points in his chapter. Each presentation was discussed by the other participants present.

Again a major goal of all present was to resolve areas of disagreement if possible. In general, the degree of agreement reached was remarkable. Contrary to expectations, areas of disagreement did *not* follow specialty orientations, but seemed to follow more conservative and less conservative spectra within specialties. At the conclusion of the oral session, all participants felt that the consensus process had been worthwhile and that the degree of agreement reached by the expert participants in the endeavor would be useful not only to them but to less expert physicians and the patients they serve throughout the world.

C. Written Documentation of the Consensus Process

This volume serves as the primary documentation of the Consensus Conference on CBAS. It includes discussions of all points of consensus or agreement, near consensus or prevailing opinion, disagreement or uncertainty. This volume also contains a chapter from 14 of the 17 consensus conference participants. These chapters summarize each participant's personal experience, current opinions, and future predictions regarding CBAS. Finally, this book contains two chapters written by the consensus conference organizers. These chapters provide the broad, current overview of CBAS that should prove valuable to all physicians as they face specific patient problems that may be best or acceptably managed by CBAS. This broad overview together with an abbreviated version of some of the other material in this volume will also be submitted to a major medical journal with all conference participants as authors.

REFERENCES

1. Tsai FY, Matovich V, Hieshima G. Percutaneous angioplasty of the carotid artery. Am J Neurorad 1986; 7:349–355.

2. Theron J, Courtheoux P, Alachkar F, Bouvard G. Maiza D. New triple coaxial catheter system for carotid angioplasty with cerebral protection. Am J Neurorad 1990; 11:869–874.

3. Matthias KD. Stent placement in complex internal carotid artery lesions (abstr). Radiol Soc N Amer 1994.

4. Yadav SJ, Roubin GS, Iyer S, et al. Elective stenting of the extracranial arteries. Circulation 1997; 95:1239–1245.

5. Wholey MH, Wholey M, Bergeron P, Diethrich EB. Henry M, LaBorde JC, et al. Current global status of carotid artery stent placement. Cathet Cardiovasc Diagn 1998; 44:1–6.

6. Diethrich EB, Ndiaye M, Reid DB. Stenting in the carotid artery: initial experience in 119 patients. J Endcvasc Surg 1996; 3:42–62.

7. Naylor AR, Bolia A, Abbott RJ, Pye IF, Smith J, Leonard N, Lloyd AJ, London NJ, Bell PR. Randomized study of carotid angioplasty and stenting versus carotid endarterectomy: a stopped trial. J Vasc Surg 1998; 28:326–334.

8. Mathur A, Roubin GS, Iyer SS, Piamsonboon C, Liu MW, Gomez CR, et al. Predictors of stroke complicating carotid artery stenting. Circulation 1998; 97:1239–1245.

9. Henry M, Amor M, Masson I, Henry I, Tzueranov K, Chati Z, Khanna N. Angioplasty and stenting of the extracranial carotid arteries. J Endovasc Surg 1998; 5:293–304.

10. Beebe HG, Archie JP, Baker WH, Barnes RW, Becker GJ, Bernstein EF, et al. Concern about safety of carotid angioplasty. Stroke 1996; 27:197–198.

11. Bettmann MA, Katzen BT, Whisnant J, Brant-Zawadzki CM, Broderick JP, Furlan AJ. Carotid stenting and angioplasty: a statement for healthcare professionals from the councils of cardiovascular radiology, stroke, cardiothoracic and vascular surgery, epidemiology and prevention, and clinical cardiology, American Heart Association. Stroke 1998; 29: 336–348.

2
Results of Consensus Questionnaire and Consensus Conference

Frank J. Veith
Montefiore Medical Center–Albert Einstein College of Medicine, New York, New York

Max Amor
U.C.C.I. Polyclinique d'Essey, Essey-les-Nancy, France

I. DEFINITIONS

All 17 consensus participants answered all 18 questions completely. Answers were collated and analyzed according to the following definitions. If *12 or more* of the 17 responding participants agreed on a response to a question about CBAS, that answer was considered to represent *consensus or general agreement*. If *10 or 11* of the 17 respondents agreed on a response, that response was considered to represent *near consensus or prevailing opinion*. Near consensus was also reached when nine respondents agreed on a response while two or three were uncertain and five or six disagreed. If only *nine or less* of the 17 participants agreed on a response to a question, that response was considered an area of *divided opinion, disagreement, or uncertainty*.

II. OVERALL RESULTS OF QUESTIONNAIRE
AND CONFERENCE

Of the 18 questions originally posed to the conference participants, consensus or agreement with regard to the answer was attained on nine, and near consensus or prevailing opinion on six. The answers to the three remaining original questions reflected divided opinion or wide ranges of opinion, based on conflicting views, uncertainty, or actual disagreement. In addition, at the oral session two derivative or altered questions were posed. With these minor alterations in the question, the answers were converted from "prevailing opinion" to consensus. Thus, consensus was reached on 11 of 20, or 55%, of the answers to key questions posed, and near consensus was reached on six of 20, or 30% of the answers.

Only in the answers to three of the 20, or 15%, of the questions was there a wide range of divergent opinions. These overall results reflect a remarkable degree of agreement among the experts on this controversial topic.

Definitions

---

17 respondents

$\geq 12/17$ = Consensus (agreement)

$10-11/17$ = Prevailing opinion (near consensus)

(or 9 + 2–3 uncertains)

$\leq 9/17$ = Divided opinion/disagreement/uncertainty

III. SPECIFIC RESULTS OF QUESTIONS TO WHICH PARTICIPANTS' RESPONSES REFLECTED CONSENSUS OR AGREEMENT

A. Should CBAS Currently Undergo Widespread Practice (i.e., Be Standard of Care)?

Of the 17 respondents, 14 answered no. Two others who voted yes would advocate use of CBAS only for specific indications or surgically unfit patients. Otherwise these two participants, one a radiologist and one a surgeon, would have voted no. Thus clear consensus was reached that *CBAS should not currently be recommended for widespread practice, i.e., become the standard of care.*

B. Should Widespread (i.e., Standard of Care) CBAS Await Results of Randomized Studies?

Of the 17 participants, 12 answered yes. One respondent, a radiologist, would vote yes if the question was not applied to high-risk patients for whom he deemed registries to be adequate. Thus, consensus was reached that *widespread application of CBAS should await the results of randomized prospective trials.*

C. Is CBAS Currently Appropriate Only for Low-Risk (NASCET-Eligible) Patients?

Of the 17 participants, 16 answered no. Thus, clear consensus was reached that *CBAS should not currently be consid-*

ered appropriate only for low-risk patients. Parenthetically one respondent commented that the CREST Trial should be performed only after high-risk registry results were available.

D. Must High-Level Neurointerventional Skills and Techniques Be Available to Perform CBAS?

Of the 17 participants, 12 answered yes; three (two cardiologists and one surgeon) answered no; and two (surgeons) were uncertain. One surgeon commented that the skills and techniques need not be possessed by the CBAS operator, but should be available within the same institution. Thus consensus was reached that *high-level neuro rescue skills and techniques must currently be available to perform CBAS.*

E. Is the Optimal Stent for Use in CBAS Currently Defined?

Of the 17 participants, 13 answered no; one surgeon answered yes; and three (two radiologists and one surgeon) indicated uncertainty. Thus *consensus was reached that the optimal stent for use in CBAS was not currently defined.*

Despite this, one cardiologist commented that current stents were adequate and one surgeon commented that nitinol stents will probably replace stainless steel stents.

F. Assuming Comparable Immediate and Late Results Between CBAS and Carotid Endarterectomy (CEA), Should CBAS Be Offered to Patients in Some Circumstances?

Of the 17 participants, 14 answered yes. Three respondents (one radiologist and two surgeons) answered no. However, four respondents acknowledged that there were currently no data to justify the assumption implied in this question. Nevertheless, consensus was reached that, *if the assumption of equivalent results for CBAS and CEA could be shown, then CBAS should be offered to patients in some circumstances.*

G. Would You Offer CBAS to Patients in All Possible Circumstances in Which Treatment of Carotid Stenosis Was Indicated?

Of the 17 participants, 13 answered no. Thus consensus was reached that *CBAS should not be offered to patients requiring treatment of carotid bifurcation stenosis in all circumstances.* Three respondents commented that this could only be done when validated data were available to justify such practice.

H. In What Circumstance Is CBAS Presently Justified in Experienced Centers?

Consensus was reached on five *presently justifiable indications for CBAS in patients requiring treatment for carotid bifurcation stenoses.* These were:

1. High-risk symptomatic patients
2. Recurrent stenosis
3. Previous radical neck dissection or cervical irradiation
4. High bifurcation or extent of the carotid lesion
5. Indications for CEA, but patient unfit for surgery

In addition, the prevailing opinion (eight of 12 of those present at the oral session) was that CBAS was also justified in patients with indications for CEA in the presence of a contralateral internal carotid occlusion. A minority (four of 12) participants, whose experience showed minimally increased risk of CEA in this circumstance, believed that this was not an indication for CBAS.

I. What Conditions Currently Contraindicate CBAS?

Consensus was reached on *five current contraindications.* These were:

1. Intraluminal thrombus
2. Complex bifurcation lesions, i.e., long, multifocal lesion or an angulated internal carotid artery
3. Extensive aortic or brachiocephalic trunk plaque; severe tortuosity or calcification of the aortic arch vessels
4. Ring-like heavy calcification of the carotid bifurcation
5. Neurologically unstable patient or a stroke within 3 weeks of the intended CBAS

Young patients (<65 or <55 years of age) were also considered by some participants to be poor candidates for CBAS, but this contraindication was felt to be inappropriate by a majority who attended the oral session.

Consensus was also reached by participants at the oral session on two modified original questions that had been posed. Answers to the original questions were consistent with near consensus or prevailing opinion. However, a number of participants altered their answers with the modified questions to produce consensus. The modified questions and their consensus answers were as follows:

J. When Cerebral Protection Devices Are Available, Should CBAS Only Be Performed with Some Form of Such Device?

All 12 of the oral session participants agreed (clear consensus) that *when cerebral protection devices were available, they should be used for CBAS.* However, three participants acknowledged that the value of these devices in lowering the incidence of periprocedural stroke has not been proven conclusively. The remaining participants believed that current evidence was adequate to mandate use of these devices when they are available.

K. Are Adequate Stents and Technology for Performing CBAS Currently Available, if Cerebral Protection Devices Were Available and Effective?

Of the 17 participants, 12 answered this question yes. Four answered no and three were uncertain. Thus consensus was reached that *adequate stents and technology are currently available for performing CBAS, when effective cerebral protection devices become available.*

IV. SPECIFIC RESULTS OF QUESTIONS TO WHICH PARTICIPANTS' RESPONSES REFLECTED NEAR CONSENSUS OR PREVAILING OPINION

A. Are the Optimal Techniques for Performing CBAS Currently Defined?

Of the 17 participants 11 answered no; and six answered yes. Thus, the prevailing opinion was that *optimal techniques for performing CBAS are not currently defined.* One cardiologist commented that this was a technique in evolution. One radiologist indicated the need for more dedicated designs of stents and introducer devices for CBAS.

B. Is CBAS Currently Appropriate for High-Risk Patients Only?

Of the 17 participants, 11 answered yes; six answered no. Thus the prevailing opinion was that *CBAS was currently appropriate only for high-risk patients.* Conceivably some of the respondents who voted no did so because they felt that CBAS should not be limited only to high-risk patients. If that were the case it would only strengthen the prevailing opinion that CBAS was currently appropriate for high-risk patients.

One surgeon commented that there was, however, a need to define high-risk patients precisely. The affirmative answers to this question were given by four radiologists, one cardiologist, and six surgeons. The negative answers were by three radiologists, two cardiologists, and one surgeon. Thus the prevailing opinion was expressed across specialty lines.

C. Is CBAS Currently Appropriate for High- and Low-Risk Patients?

Of the 17 participants, 10 answered this question no; five answered yes; and two were uncertain. Thus, the prevailing opinion was that *CBAS is not currently appropriate for high- and low-risk patients.*

Of the 10 affirmative answers, three were given by radiologists, one by a cardiologist, and six by surgeons. Thus again the prevailing opinion was expressed across specialty lines. The two uncertain answers were expressed by radiologists who felt that clinical trials were needed to define indications precisely.

D. For CBAS Operators with Complication Rates Equal to or Better Than Guidelines for CEA, Should They Presently Be Able to Offer Their Patients a Carotid Stenting Option?

Of the 17 participants, 11 answered this question yes; six answered no. Three of the individuals who answered negatively commented that there was insufficient valid comparative data in comparable patients to justify an affirmative answer. This lack of data was particularly evident with regard to late results. Nevertheless, the prevailing opinion was that *CBAS operators with complication rates equivalent*

to those for CEA should presently be able to offer some pa-
tients a stenting option. Again this prevailing opinion was
expressed by individuals from all three specialties (five radiologists, three cardiologists, and three surgeons).

E. Should CBAS Currently Only Be Performed with Some Form of Cerebral Protection Device?

Of the 17 participants, nine answered this question no; five
answered yes; and three were uncertain. Thus, the prevailing opinion was that *CBAS currently can be performed with-*
out a cerebral protection device. It should be noted, however, that the European respondents largely answered yes
to this question probably because such devices are available to them. On the other hand, U.S. respondents tended
to answer no because such devices are not presently available in the United States. It is also noteworthy that three
participants (one radiologist, two surgeons) considered the
value of cerebral protection devices unproven.

When the question was modified slightly [at the oral
session (see above)], clear consensus was reached that
CBAS should only be performed with some form of cerebral
protection device when such a device is available.

F. Are Adequate Stents and Technology for Performing CBAS Currently Available?

Of the 17 participants, 10 answered yes; four answered no;
and three were uncertain. Thus, the prevailing opinion was
that *adequate stents and technology for performing CBAS*
are currently available. That opinion was expressed across
specialty lines (four radiologists, two cardiologists, and four
surgeons). When the question was slightly modified at the
oral session to assume that effective cerebral protection devices were available, a consensus affirmative answer to this
question was obtained (see above).

V. SPECIFIC RESULTS OF QUESTIONS TO WHICH PARTICIPANTS' RESPONSES REFLECTED DIVIDED OPINION, DISAGREEMENT, OR UNCERTAINTY

A. Should an FDA Investigational Device Exemption (IDE) Be Required to Perform CBAS in the United States, or Should Comparable Approval Be Required Elsewhere?

Of the 17 participants, nine answered no and eight yes. Thus *opinion on this question was clearly divided.* One surgeon commented that an IDE should be required except for an occasional case. One radiologist commented that IDEs should only be required during clinical trials. Of interest was the specialty alignment of the participants. The eight affirmative answers were from three radiologists, one cardiologist, and four surgeons; the nine negative answers were from four radiologists, two cardiologists, and three surgeons. Thus there was no specialty bias for either answer.

B. What Proportion of Patients Requiring Treatment for Carotid Bifurcation Disease Are Presently Acceptable for CBAS?

The 17 participants had a wide range of proposed percentages in answer to this question. These divergent opinions ranged from <5% to approximately 100% with a mean of 44%. There was also a wide range of overlapping answers within each specialty, although the highest responses (>60%) were in the answers of the interventional specialists. Radiologists' answers were <5%, 6%, 15%, 80%, 90%, approximately 100%, and uncertain (mean 49%). Cardiologists' answers were 40%, 80%, and 95% (mean 72%). Surgeons answers were 5%, 10%, 20%, 20%, 35%, 60%, and uncertain (mean 25%).

C. What Proportion of Patients Requiring Treatment for Carotid Bifurcation Disease Are Presently Best or Optimally Treated by CBAS?

Again the 17 participants had a wide range of proposed percentages in answer to this question. These divergent opinions ranged from <3% to approximately 100% with a mean of 34%. Again there was a wide range of overlapping answers within each specialty. Radiologists' answers were 3%, <5%, 15%, 45%, 90%, approximately 100%, and uncertain (mean 43%). Cardiologists' answers were 25%, 80%, and uncertain (mean 53%). Surgeons' answers were <3%, <5%, 5%, 15%, 20%, 25%, and 50% (mean 18%).

3

Defining the High-Risk Carotid Endarterectomy Patient

Implications for Carotid Angioplasty and Stenting Trials

Hugh G. Beebe
University of Michigan Medical School, Ann Arbor, Michigan, and Jobst Vascular Center, Toledo, Ohio

As is always true in the application of new and evolving technology, a debate arises over appropriate use of the new approach in early clinical experience. In the case of carotid disease treatment with the goal of preventing stroke, many factors have served to heighten the intensity of the debate over early application of carotid angioplasty and stenting.

This discussion will examine evidence regarding factors that have been used to identify patients at higher than average risk for carotid endarterectomy to see if it makes sense to apply them as justification for clinical investigation of the new catheter-based treatment. But first, let's begin with a brief listing of influences that have heightened the debate about carotid stenting, if only to frame a background for considering how to define the higher-risk patient.

Factors that have made the discussion about carotid angioplasty and stenting appear contentious include:

1. Its introduction immediately following reporting of best-quality randomized trials of carotid endarterectomy
2. Its application generally by specialists who were not vascular surgeons or surgeons who did carotid surgery and thus were new to the field
3. Relative paucity of data regarding both early and late outcomes
4. Reporting standards that made precise interpretation of results difficult
5. Early widespread inclusion in continuing medical education programs that appeared to promote interest in application of a technique at an investigational stage
6. Widespread perception that the technology was evolving and unsettled, e.g., stent types, embolism trapping devices
7. A background of persistently unsettled indications for treatment of the asymptomatic patient with carotid stenosis by surgery or any method
8. Intuitive concerns based on assumptions about endovascular manipulation of the carotid atheroma

These and other factors often have left the dialogue about clinical use of carotid angioplasty and stenting in the realm of opinion, sometimes accompanied by emotion, but relatively little data.

I. BACKGROUND OF RISK ASSESSMENT IN CAROTID SURGERY

Risk evaluation in surgical decisions is easiest when making a relative comparison between the risk of a treatment versus the risk of the condition's natural history without such treatment. But, that is not what is being considered here. When risk between two treatment alternatives is being considered, the process is often difficult because of unequal data available for comparison and complex personal bias on the part of both doctor and patient. There is no better example of how difficult this process can be than comparing carotid endarterectomy and carotid stenting.

For example, even though the long-term results of endograft for abdominal and thoracic aneurysm are not yet known, the short-term benefits are sufficiently compelling that many doctors and patients prefer the endovascular treatment. A good part of that bias derives from the great difference in physiological cost between conventional open surgery versus less invasive endografts.

But, carotid endarterectomy is not a very big operation, many patients going home in 24–36 hr these days, so the physiological cost difference between endarterectomy and angioplasty and stenting is minimal. Thus it makes sense to put great emphasis and value on attempting to identify a subset of patients at higher-than-average risk for endarterectomy because using a new procedure becomes more rational in such a group.

This discussion considers several questions: 1) Can a "high risk" surgical (carotid endarterectomy) subset be identified? 2) How strong is the evidence supporting that

Table 1   Risk Factors in Carotid Endarterectomy

Advanced age
Contralateral carotid occlusion
Contralateral severe carotid stenosis
Vertebral artery stenosis
Severe intracranial carotid tandem stenosis
High carotid bifurcation
Recurrent stenosis
Prior history of stroke
Unstable neurological symptoms
Renal failure
Diabetes mellitus

perception of risk? 3) Are there confounding factors that make classifying risk difficult to generalize?

II. IDENTIFYING HIGH-RISK FACTORS

For purposes of this discussion, "risk" means the risk of stroke or death. There are other important risks such as myocardial infarction and a long list of nonspecific surgical complications that are not considered for practical reasons. Many factors that have been nominated as increasing carotid endarterectomy (CEA) risk are summarized in Table 1.

III. HOW STRONG IS THE EVIDENCE?

A. Advanced Age

Elderly patients have been called a high-risk group for carotid endarterectomy because age has generally increased risk of most surgical procedures and because the carotid stenting literature often has made a point of basing risk assessment on the NASCET (North American Symptomatic Carotid Endarterectomy Trial) criteria, which include age limitation. Is this borne out by the data?

Perler and Williams (1) reported a 4.8% perioperative stroke and death rate in 59 patients aged ≥75 years having CEA during the interval 1982–1994. Two-year follow up on 54 patients showed a rate of 92% cumulative freedom from stroke. The authors concluded the CEA is justified in elderly patients and excellent long-term results can be achieved. Treiman et al. (2) reviewed 146 patients 80 years of age or older having 183 CEA from 1964 to 1990 with an aggregate total of three strokes (1.6%) and three deaths (1.6%), 3.2% total. Also, 28 (19%) of their octogenarian cohort had a history of prior stroke. They recommended that similar evaluation criteria for CEA be applied to all patients, regardless of age, but that the indication for operation among asymptomatic elderly patients should be more conservative than that used for younger patients.

In 1984–1985, Fisher and colleagues (3) reviewed Medicare data for 2089 patients over age 65 and found all-cause mortality after CEA increased proportionately with age. The risk of death within 30 days of CEA was 1.1% for ages 65–69, 2.8% for ages 70–74, 3.2% for ages 75–79, and 4.7% for those over age 80. In a similar study of 113,300 Medicare patients undergoing CEA in 1992 and 1993, the same authors found comparable results (4). The perioperative mortality rate was 1.2% for ages 65–69, 1.46% for ages 70–74, 1.98% for ages 75–79, 2.46% for ages 80–84, and 3.6% for patients ≥85 years. Another population-based study of Medicare patients was reported by Richardson and Main (5), who found a combined stroke and death rate of 4.3% in patients over age 65 with a mean age of 71 years. But for those with asymptomatic lesions the rate was only 2.8%.

The University of Rochester, an institution with particular interest in carotid artery disease, reported a 3.9%

stroke rate (0 deaths) in 77 CEA performed in patients over 75 years and also that this was not different from the 3.1% stroke rate among 470 patients less than that age (6). This report was from experience in the early 1980s.

More recently two reports document contemporary results. Ballotta et al. (7) had 0% strokes and death in 96 patients over age 75 having 103 CEAs. O'Hara et al. (8) at the Cleveland Clinic Foundation performed 182 CEAs in 167 patients aged 80 or above. There were three strokes (1.6%) and one death (0.6%).

The mean combined stroke and death rate of eight papers each reporting CEA in more than 50 patients aged 75 or above was 3.8%. Taken together, it seems incorrect to assign much influence to age per se in determination of risk for operative stroke and death in carotid surgery.

B. Systemic Comorbidity

From January 1990 to December 1995, LoGerfo and colleagues (9) at the New England Deaconess Hospital, a center for diabetes care, performed 284 CEAs in patients with diabetes out of a total of 732 CEAs. They found that patients with diabetes fared no worse. After CEA there was a 1.0% stroke and 0.35% death rate in patients with diabetes and 1.1% and 0.2% rates, respectively, among those without diabetes. The same group (10) studied the effect of renal failure on CEA risk and found a 1.18% stroke and death rate among those with creatinine < 1.5 mg/dL ($n = 928$) but 6.94% in those with all degrees of renal failure ($n = 73$).

Goldstein et al. (11), from Duke University's Center for Health Policy Research and Education, assessed risk factors among 697 patients having CEA for lesions with ipsilateral symptoms. The following risk factors were *not* a significant influence on complication rates: gender, race, age > 75 years, myocardial infarction within 6 months, congestive heart failure, chronic obstructive pulmonary disease, severe hypertension, angina, contralateral carotid stenosis or occlusion, or angiographic evidence of ulcer.

C. Cerebrovascular Anatomy

The status of collateral blood supply has been examined as an influence on CEA results for many years and recently advocated as an indication for stenting because of reduced occlusion time during the procedure. Modern publications have emphasized that contralateral occlusion does not show an adverse result of outcomes, however.

Ballota et al. (12) reported two strokes (3.5%) and one death (1.7%) in 57 CEA patients with contralateral occlusion (only 63% shunted), which was not significantly different from three strokes (1%) and two deaths (0.7%) in 279 patients with patent contralateral internal carotid arteries. Surgeons at Emory University (13) found that a 4.3% 30-day combined stroke and death rate in 116 patients with contralateral carotid occlusion was not different from a 4.0% rate among 956 patients without contralateral occlusion. Intraluminal shunts were used in 115 cases.

At New York University, another institution with long-standing special expertise in carotid disease, an interesting report (14) compared patients with contralateral occlusion having CEA in two different time periods. Among 180 patients treated in 1965–1984 the perioperative stroke and death rate was 6.7%. But in 135 patients treated by CEA from 1985 to 1991 this rate dropped to 0.7%. The increased use of shunting in the latter group (29% to 52%) did not alone account for the improved results.

Vertebral artery occlusive disease was associated with an increased stroke and death rate after CEA, 19/306 (6.2%), compared to those having CEA without vertebral artery involvement, 23/1001 (2.3%) ($p = 0.003$), in a large German study (15). Whether this was a specific influence or perhaps a marker for diffuse cerebrovascular disease was not clear.

D. The Carotid Lesion Itself

An uncontrolled, but theoretically reasonable dictum of carotid surgery has been the importance of limited, gentle
handling of the carotid artery during exposure to avoid embolism, especially in the presence of an ulcerated atheroma. However, results do not seem to support lesion ulceration as a risk factor. As a matter of fact, the identification
of ulceration by angiography is poor. The most thorough
study available from examination of NASCET results in 500
patients who had prospective angiographic ulcer detection
compared with surgical specimen histology showed only a
sensitivity of 45.9% and specificity of 74.1% regardless of
the degree of stenosis (16).

Still further interesting evidence on this issue comes
from both preoperative computed tomography (CT) evidence of cerebral infarction and transcranial Doppler study
during CEA. Blohme et al. (17) found that presence of CT
signs of cerebral infarction significantly increased risk from
2.8% stroke or death rate without cerebral infarction to
9.8% for all those with cerebral infarction signs on CT X-
rays ($p = 0.008$). Many other factors, such as use of shunts,
operative and postoperative blood pressure, and adjunctive
neuromedications, influence this issue and can be pre-
sumed to be more important in patients with evidence of
previous cerebral infarction.

When transcranial Doppler was used by Levi et al. (18)
during CEA, microembolic signals were detected in 94% of
patients intraoperatively. But this factor per se had no influence on the operative stroke and death rate. Gaunt and
colleagues (19) at the Leicester Royal Infirmary found
transcranial Doppler evidence of intraprocedural embolization during CEA in 92% of 100 consecutive, monitored patients, but no association with adverse clinical outcome.
Observations in this study included neurological examination, psychometric testing, fundoscopy with automated
field defect testing, and CT brain scans.

In the study by Goldstein et al. (11), there was a strong trend in favor of increased risk associated with intraluminal thrombus and carotid siphon stenosis that appeared to be statistically significant.

E. Reoperation for Carotid Stenosis

Although previously accepted carotid surgery standards have recognized an increased risk in CEA for recurrent stenosis (20), recent studies of this indication for CEA have concluded that operation for recurrent stenosis is as safe and effective as primary CEA and should continue to be the standard treatment. Hill and colleagues (21) at Stanford University Medical Center reported no deaths and no strokes (and no cranial nerve injuries) among 40 consecutive CEAs for recurrent stenosis compared to a 1.1% stroke and death rate for 350 primary operations in the same time period.

IV. CONFOUNDING FACTORS THAT MAKE CLASSIFYING RISK DIFFICULT TO GENERALIZE

It is difficult to objectively describe technical expertise that resides in a particular environment comprised of physicians and surgeons with special interest in carotid artery disease and highly skilled supporting staffs within their institution. But it is likely that this factor influences results of CEA.

Riles et al. (22) thoughtfully examined the cause of perioperative stroke among 3,062 CEAs performed in 2365 patients during the period 1965–1991. They concluded that among the 66 patients with perioperative stroke, 2.2% overall and 1.5% during the last 5-year interval, most were caused by technical errors made during surgery and thus theoretically preventable. This remarkably low, but not unique, rate for all indications in a referral institution calls into question the simplistic notion of assigning the designation of "high risk" for carotid endarterectomy.

This view was upheld by an intriguing study reported by Davies et al. (23), who attempted to identify a subgroup of high-risk patients by reviewing 404 CEA procedures with a 2% mortality rate, a 3.4% transient ischemic attack rate, and a 4% stroke rate. Multiple logistic regression showed no influence on outcome of age, gender, surgical indication, bilateral disease, hypertension, or smoking history. Technical factors were not examined.

V. USE OF THE NASCET CRITERIA FOR RISK STRATIFICATION

No discussion about defining the high-risk CEA patient would be complete without mentioning use of the NASCET inclusion/exclusion criteria as a risk-indexing system as they have been used in some publications in the carotid stenting literature.

Some of the NASCET criteria unquestionably do increase risk, not only for CEA, but in general terms that would apply to carotid stenting as well. For example, uncontrolled hypertension, unstable angina, progressing stroke, and uncontrolled diabetes are important predictors of morbidity, most of which ought to be controlled before attempting any form of cerebral revascularization procedure.

There are other factors that are not demonstrably associated with increased risk for CEA but were included in the NASCET selection criteria for two purposes: to increase the likelihood that the patient could be followed long enough to determine outcome at a significant interval and to increase obtaining a clear, readily interpretable end point, thus enhancing the study's chance of coming to a definitive conclusion about its results.

The usual process of establishing a risk stratification scheme for anything is to apply it first retrospectively to see if the criteria make sense for the intended purpose. Subsequently the defined criteria must be validated by prospective application to prove their worth. The NASCET study criteria were not designed for the purpose of carotid surgery risk stratification and have never been prospectively applied in such a manner to identify patients at higher risk for the operation. Thus, to use the NASCET study entry criteria inappropriately to claim risk advantages for any treatment of carotid disease seems scientifically naive and incorrect.

VI. CONCLUSIONS

Identifying patient factors that predict higher-than-average risk for carotid endarterectomy is not a finished task and may never be if one accepts the premise that operator skill and the level of hospital care are major influences on outcome. Some of the general risk factors that predict increased morbidity for any procedure will accompany carotid angioplasty and stenting interventions as well. Individual institutions could resolve the issue of identifying the "high risk" carotid patient by maintaining an ongoing registry of their results and examining all of the potentially influential risk factors in relationship to treatment outcomes. This might provide a way to determine the preferred approach for specific patients using local evidence-based decision making.

REFERENCES

1. Perler BA, Williams GM. Carotid endarterectomy in the very elderly: is it worthwhile? Surgery 1994; 116:479–483.
2. Treiman RL, Wagner WH, Foran RF, Cossman DV, Levin PM, Cohen JL, Treiman GS. Carotid endarterectomy in the elderly. Ann Vasc Surg 1992; 6:321–324.

3. Fisher ES, Malenka DJ, Solomon NA, Bubolz TA, Whaley FS, Wennberg JE. Risk of carotid endarterectomy in the elderly. Am J Public Health 1989; 79:1617–1620.

4. Wennberg DE, Lucas FL, Birkmeyer JD, Bredenberg CE, Fisher ES. Variation in carotid endarterectomy mortality in the Medicare population. Trial hospitals, volume, and patient characteristics. JAMA 1998; 279:1278–1281.

5. Richardson JD, Main KA. Carotid endarterectomy in the elderly population: a statewide experience. J Vasc Surg 1989; 9:65–73.

6. Ouriel K, Penn TE, Ricotta JJ, May AG, Green RM, DeWeese JA. Carotid endarterectomy in the elderly patient. Surg Gynecol Obstet 1986; 162:334–336.

7. Ballotta E, Da Giau G, Saladini M, Abbruzzese E. Carotid endarterectomy in symptomatic and asymptomatic patients aged 75 years or more: perioperative mortality and stroke risk rates. Ann Vasc Surg 1999; 13:158–163.

8. O'Hara PJ, Hertzer NR, Mascha EJ, Beven EG, Krajewski LP, Sullivan TM. Carotid endarterectomy in octogenarians: early results and late outcome. J Vasc Surg 1998; 27:860–871.

9. Akbari CM, Pomposelli FB Jr, Gibbons GW, Campbell DR, Freeman DV, LoGerfo FW. Diabetes mellitus: a risk factor for carotid endarterectomy? J Vasc Surg 1997; 25:1070–1076.

10. Hamdan AD, Pomposelli FB Jr, Gibbons GW, Campbell DR, LoGerfo FW. Renal insufficiency and altered postoperative risk in carotid endarterectomy. J Vasc Surg 1999; 29:1006–1011.

11. Goldstein LB, McCrory DC, Landsman PB, Samsa GP, Ancukiewicz M, Oddone EZ, Matchar DB. Multicenter review of preoperative risk factors for carotid endarterectomy in patients with ipsilateral symptoms. Stroke 1994; 25:1116–1121.

12. Ballotta E, Da Giau G, Guerra M. Carotid endarterectomy and contralateral internal carotid artery occlusion: perioperative risks and long-term stroke and survival rates. Surgery 1998; 123:234–240.

13. Coyle KA, Smith RB 3rd, Salam AA, Dodson TF, Chaikof EL,

Lumsden AB. Carotid endarterectomy in patients with contralateral carotid occlusion: review of a 10-year experience. Cardiovasc Surg 1996; 4:71–75.

14. Adelman MA, Jacobowitz GR, Riles TS, Imparato AM, Lamparello PJ, Baumann FG, Landis R. Carotid endarterectomy in the presence of a contralateral occlusion: a review of 315 cases over a 27-year experience. Cardiovasc Surg 1995; 3: 307–312.

15. Hoffmann A, Dinkel M, Schweiger H, Lang W. The influence of the state of the vertebral arteries on the peri- and postoperative risk in carotid surgery. Eur J Vasc Endovasc Surg 1998; 16:329–333.

16. Streifler JY, Eliasziw M, Fox AJ, Benavente OR, Hachinski VC, Ferguson GG, Barnett HJ. Angiographic detection of carotid plaque ulceration. Comparison with surgical observations in a multicenter study. North American Symptomatic Carotid Endarterectomy Trial. Stroke 1994; 25:1130–1132.

17. Blohme L, Sandstrom V, Hellstrom G, Swedenborg J, Takolander R. Complications in carotid endarterectomy are predicted by qualifying symptoms and preoperative CT findings. Eur J Vasc Endovasc Surg 1999; 17:213–218.

18. Levi CR, Roberts AK, Fell G, Hoare MC, Royle JP, Chan A, Beiles BC, Last GC, Bladin CF, Donnan GA. Transcranial Doppler microembolus detection in the identification of patients at high risk of perioperative stroke. Eur J Vasc Endovasc Surg 1997; 14:170–176.

19. Gaunt ME, Martin PJ, Smith JL, Rimmer T, Cherryman G, Ratliff DA, Bell PR, Naylor AR. Clinical relevance of intraoperative embolization detected by transcranial Doppler ultrasonography during carotid endarterectomy: a prospective study of 100 patients. Br J Surg 1994; 81:1435–1439.

20. Beebe HG, Clagett GP, DeWeese JA, Moore WS, Robertson JT, Sandok B, Wolf PA. Assessing risk associated with carotid endarterectomy. A statement for health professionals by an Ad Hoc Committee on Carotid Surgery Standards of the Stroke Council, American Heart Association. Circulation 1989; 79:472–473.

21. Hill BB, Olcott C IV, Dalman RL, Harris EJ Jr, Zarins CK.

Reoperation for carotid stenosis is as safe as primary carotid endarterectomy. J Vasc Surg 1999; 30:26–35.

22. Riles TS, Imparato AM, Jacobowitz GR, Lamparello PJ, Giangola G, Adelman MA, Landis R. The cause of perioperative stroke after carotid endarterectomy. J Vasc Surg 1994; 19: 206–216.

23. Davies AH, Hayward JK, Currie I, Cole SE, Lopatazidis A, Lamont PM, Baird RN. Risk prediction of outcome following carotid endarterectomy. Cardiovasc Surg 1996; 4:338–339.

4
Angioplasty and Stenting at the Carotid Bifurcation, Part I

Peter R. F. Bell
University of Leicester and University Hospitals of Leicester NHS Trust, Leicester Royal Infirmary, Leicester, England

Amman Bolia
University Hospitals of Leicester NHS Trust, Leicester Royal Infirmary, Leicester, England

Carotid endarterectomy is an established technique for the treatment of carotid birufcation stenosis. The postoperative stroke rate almost 10 years ago in ECST (1) and NASCET (2) trials was around 5–7%. More recent studies have, however, shown that this can be brought down to <2% in specialized centers using such techniques as local anesthesia (3), quality control during and after surgery (4), and appropriate follow-up. Angioplasty has of course been used in many arteries and it was therefore not surprising that this technique should be used for carotid artery lesions by enthusiasts (5,6), who have published results that compare favorably with the ECST and NASCET trials. These studies unfortunately failed to recognize that current angioplasty data cannot be compared with historical controls such as ECST and NASCET. The other obvious difficulty is that the ECST and NASCET trials are not only historical but also refer to symptomatic patients. Many of the reports on angioplasty contain a significant number of patients who are asymptomatic, and therefore, once again direct comparisons with surgery cannot be made.

Another difficulty is that single-center studies usually allow exclusion of cases that are considered unsuitable for angioplasty because they have excessive calcification or are said to contain intraluminal thrombus or unsuitable plaques. The problem of course is that no one can tell, using current techniques, what an unsuitable plaque is, whether calcification matters, or if thrombus is present in the lumen. This therefore allows a completely unquantifiable approach to trials where lesions that might cause a problem are often not treated. This is perfectly reasonable provided that direct comparisons are then not made between surgery and angioplasty as they usually are. Clearly some patients can be dealt with by angioplasty quite safely and these are patients with smooth lesions that are not likely to embolize during the procedure (7). Emboli are undoubtedly a problem during angioplasty and these can be large causing morbidity or mortality (7). They often cause serious strokes or psychometric changes, which have been documented. Finally, it is known from the ECST and NASCET studies that only 30% of patients who are symptomatic actually need treatment. The other 70% would do well without any intervention at all. It may be that those patients who do well from angioplasty are the ones who have relatively smooth plaques or who have a lesser degree of stenosis. This remains to be seen.

Because of these various concerns, particularly the ability to leave out patients thought to be unsuitable for angioplasty, we set out to do a randomized study based on the intention-to-treat method. In this way it was possible to make sure that those patients who we thought were bad enough for invasive treatment were randomized to angioplasty or endarterectomy without any exclusions. Thus, no bias between the cases randomized to either treatment was possible.

The trial received Ethical Committee approval for an initial 50 patients and a monitoring committee was set up to ensure that if the trial appeared to be causing harm to patients, it could be stopped.

I. INCLUSION CRITERIA

Patients were investigated by duplex alone (Fig. 1); angiography was not used in any of these cases. A decision on treatment was made during a single clinic visit, and those with ipsilateral 70–99% stenosis as determined by the ECST criteria were randomized to either CEA or CA. All patients were symptomatic over a 6-month period. Twenty-three patients were randomized to either treatment, seven to CA, and 12 to CEA; 17 were treated before the trial was suspended by the monitoring committee. All patients were assessed by duplex scanning immediately prior to surgery to ensure that the lesion had not occluded. In addition, the plaques were categorized using the Gray-Weale (8) plaque

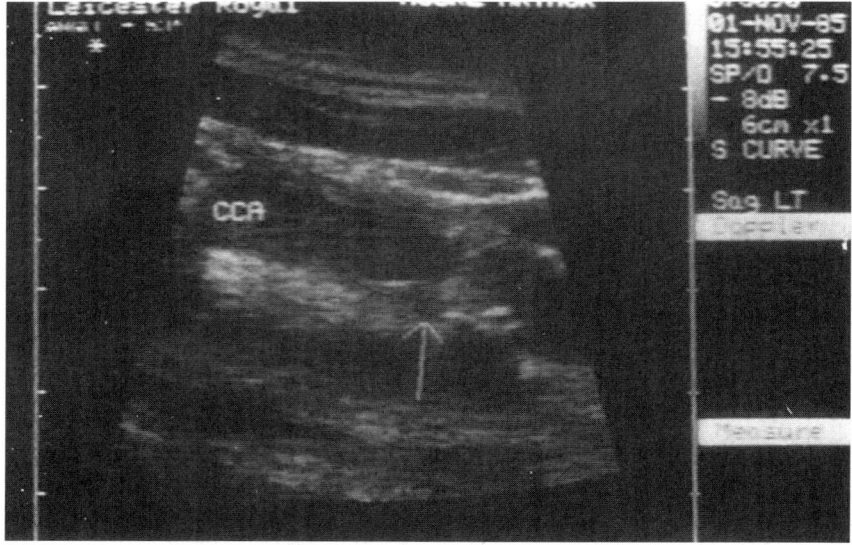

Figure 1 Duplex scan showing significant carotid stenosis.

morphology score, which allowed us to differentiate between echolucent and ulcerated plaques with thrombus. The Lusby Surface Feature Score (9) was also used to try to categorize plaques to those thought to be dangerous and those thought to be benign. All patients were examined by a consultant neurologist before and at regular intervals after the procedure was undertaken.

II. CAROTID ENDARTERECTOMY

The operation was performed without withdrawing aspirin, which all patients were taking. General anesthesia was used in all cases with loop magnification. Routine shunting using a Pruitt Inhara shunt and routine patching using Dacron was undertaken. Transcranial doppler (TCD) monitoring was used throughout the procedure to look for emboli and to assess middle cerebral blood velocity. This technique was also used to monitor the cerebral circulation for emboli for 6 hr postoperatively. This was undertaken because of evidence from our own previous studies that embolization can occur in the early postoperative period (10). All cases were examine by angioscopy prior to completion of the patch to ensure there were no technical errors. Any patient who had evidence of more than 25 emboli during any 10-min period postoperatively was given intravenous dextran 40 initially at a dose of 20 mL/hr increasing to 40 mL/hr if the embolization did not stop. Patients were followed up after endarterectomy at 1 and 3 months using duplex to assess the operation site.

III. ANGIOPLASTY

The consultant radiologist undertaking this technique had experience in more than 5000 angioplasties in peripheral

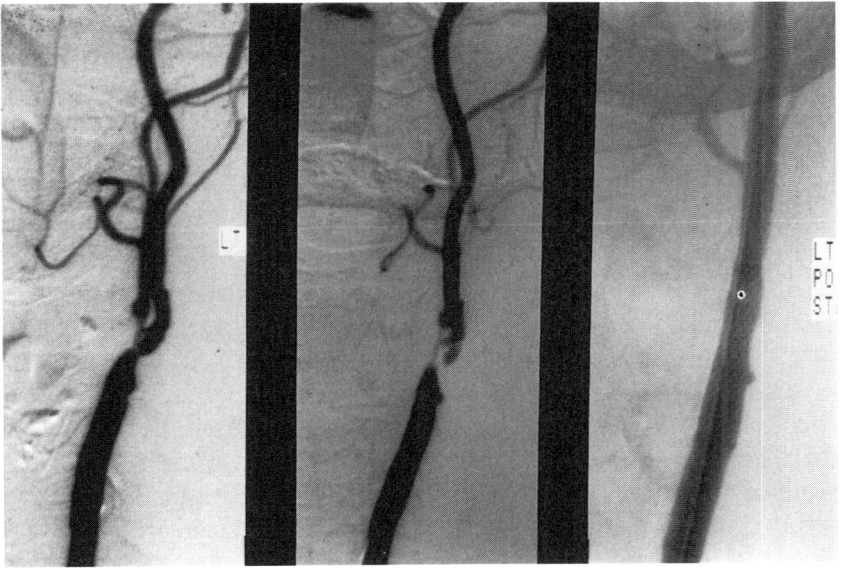

Figure 2 Carotid stenosis before and after insertion of the stent.

arteries in every part of the body. In addition, he had performed eight angioplasties in selected patients who had recurrent carotid stenoses and carotid bifurcation disease. He had also visited one of the pioneers of angioplasty (11) and was tutored by him prior to undertaking this study. The common femoral artery was cannulated using the Seldinger technique and the guidewire was passed into the aortic arch; the common carotid artery was then cannulated with a hydrophilic guidewire followed by a vertebral catheter to allow angiography and road mapping. Heparin 5000 units was given along with 600 µg atropine prior to balloon inflation. The stent size was calculated from the angiogram and the technique practiced by Matthias (11) was used to insert the stent. If any resistance was felt when the stent approached the stenosis, predilatation using a 4-mm balloon was undertaken. This was followed by the insertion of a self-expanding Schneider wall stent (Fig. 2). After deployment the stent was dilated usually with a 6-mm balloon. A completion angiogram was performed thereafter. Throughout the procedure TCD monitoring was undertaken and continued for 6 hr after the procedure was completed.

IV. RESULTS

There were no complications in those patients undergoing carotid endarterectomy and all were discharged on day 5. There were no deaths within 30 days. The patients undergoing carotid angioplasty had a number of problems, which are listed in Table 1. Of seven patients five had strokes, three of which were disabling, at 30 days. During the procedure large numbers of emboli were detected during the passage of the guidewire (Fig. 3), dilatation with a balloon, and stent deployment (Fig. 4) and are summarized in Table 2. Because of these complications, the trial was stopped by the monitoring committee. None of these patients with epi-

Table 1 Results of Carotid Angioplasty

Sex	Age (years)	Presentation	Degree of stenosis (%)	Complications
M	63	Stroke	75	None
F	57	Stroke	80	None
M	78	TIA	90	CVA
F	68	Stroke	95	Mild stroke
M	72	Amaurosis	70	CVA
M	70	TIA	90	CVA
M	74	Stroke	80	CVA

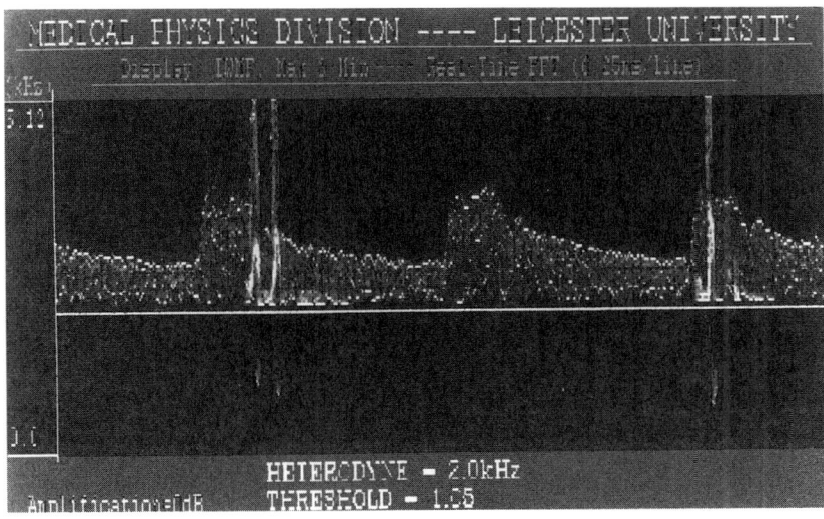

Figure 3 Emboli detected on TCD during passage of the guidewire.

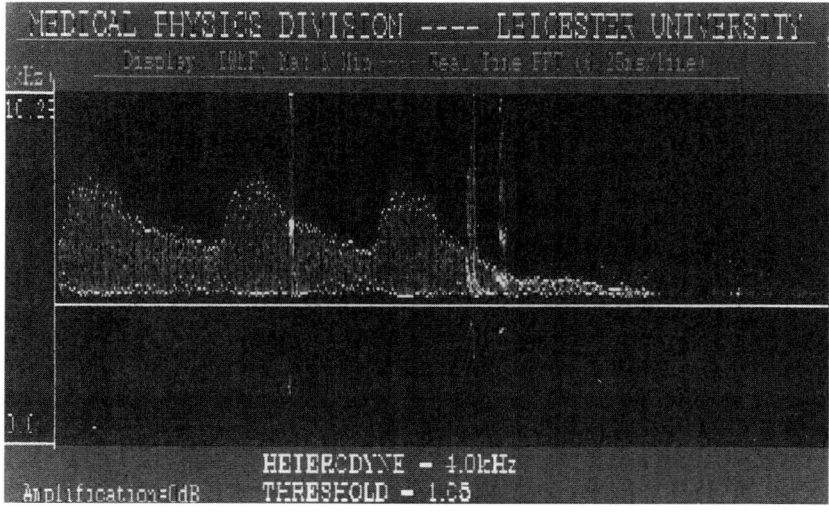

Figure 4 Emboli seen on TCD during balloon inflation of the stent.

sodes of stroke has recovered significantly since the end of the trial.

V. DISCUSSION

This study has differed from all other studies where carotid angioplasty has been used in that no patients were excluded. All other studies have not been properly randomized allowing a number of exclusions for calcification and supposed thrombus inside the vessel, ulceration, etc. Usually, therefore, the more serious cases have been dealt with by surgical treatment. As a result comparisons cannot be drawn between these two treatments. Even the recently completed CAVATAS study, which was randomized, had a number of escape clauses that allowed exclusion of patients from angioplasty if the lesions were considered unsuitable in an undefined and unquantifiable fashion (12).

Table 2 Number of Emboli Detected During Carotid Angioplasty

Time of detection of emboli	Number of emboli						
	Case 1	Case 2	Case 3	Case 4	Case 5	Case 6	Case 7
Manipulation of wire across stenosis	29	20	115	50	71	158	115
Balloon predilatation	0	56	21	0	60	42	1
Stent deployment	125	90	110	65	159	76	115
Balloon inflation	1	28	23	14	29	0	0
Balloon deflation	26	81	101	22	60	86	53
Total emboli	181	275	370	151	379	362	284
OHS stroke score at 30 days	No CVA	No CVA	3	0	2	3	3

Even then the angioplasty group stroke and death rate was more than 10.3% which was the same as that experienced by the surgeons. Unfortunately this study did not comply with the Consort Document (13) and means very little because of the exclusions and the lack of knowledge of those who were not treated.

What conclusions can be drawn from all of this? From our own experience, angioplasty in unselected patients is unacceptable because of the morbidity, which is too high compared with carotid endarterectomy. Unquestionably this is due to the production of large numbers of emboli, which is hardly a surprise when the lesions being dealt with are considered (Fig. 5). Until emboli can be controlled, the procedure should be regarded as unsafe in any patient with severe stenosis. By contrast CEA, if undertaken in a controlled environment and with quality control measures in place, can produce excellent results. Until angioplasty can equal this safety record it should not be used widely. The arrival of new protection devices including a balloon incor-

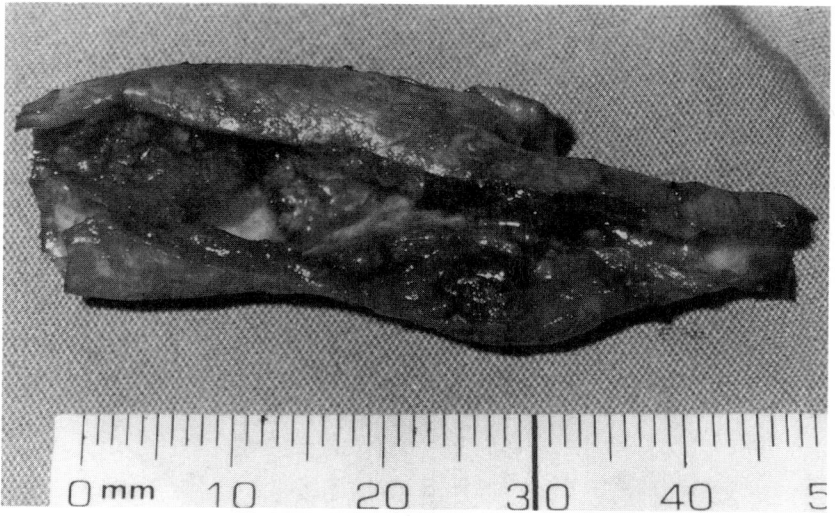

Figure 5 A severe carotid lesion.

porated into a thin wire (PercuSurge) and umbrellas that allow flow to continue (AngioGuard) (14) may well allow better results to be obtained in the future. The insertion of these thin, .014-in. devices on a guidewire system may allow minimal embolization and retrieval of embolic material during angioplasty thereby preventing the ill effects currently seen without protection.

Clearly the discussion about angioplasty versus surgery will arise repeatedly unless a proper randomized controlled trial is performed. If this is to be done, a number of issues need to be addressed before such a trial can be started. For example, should all patients who are now suitable for CEA be randomized? Are there any criteria by which patients can be selected safely for CA? Can we tell what is a safe lesion? Should CA be confined to lesions that are less severely stenosed, i.e., 70–85% in diameter stenosis? Should an asymptomatic patient be treated at all? Should balloon-expandable stents be used in view of the possibility of collapse of these stents and should the procedure be limited to only those centers that have a large throughput of cases?

Embolization undoubtedly occurs during the passage of a wire and all stages of carotid angioplasty (Table 2). For this reason to do a trial without using protection devices is in our opinion, unacceptable. The trial perhaps should be done in a staged fashion, the initial project being to compare patients who have stenoses of 70–85% without calcification, ulceration, or thrombus. Bearing in mind that you cannot tell whether thrombus or ulceration is present in every case, this will in itself be difficult. If this study shows no difference between surgery and angioplasty, the next stage could be approached and more difficult cases dealt with.

A number of issues are not being examined critically and these would include restenosis within a stent in the carotid artery, which in our practice is a significant problem not only in the carotid artery but in other areas as well. It may be that we have to do other trials in the future to look at ways of stopping this happening, such as brachytherapy or the incorporation of drugs on the stent when these become available. Only if a proper study is done without any exclusion clauses, which compares like with like, will we be able to really discover the role that carotid angioplasty has to play in the treatment of this common condition. We suspect that if research is concentrated to try to find those patients who actually need treatment, the dangerous ones are better dealt with by surgery or angioplasty if that can be shown to be comparable.

REFERENCES

1. European Carotid Surgery Trialists Collaborative Group. MRC European Carotid Surgery Trial. Interim Results for Symptomatic Patients with severe (70–99%) or with mild (0–29%) carotid stenosis. Lancet 1991; 337:1235–1243.
2. North American Symptomatic Carotid Endarterectomy Trial Collaborators. Beneficial effect of carotid endarterectomy in symptomatic patients with high grade score in stenosis. N Engl J Med 1991; 325:445–453.
3. Shah DM, Darling C III, Chenby B, et al. Carotid endarterectomy in awake patients: safety, acceptability and outcome. J Vasc Surg 1994; 19:1015–1020.
4. Naylor AR, Gaunt ME. Quality control during carotid endarterectomy. Vasc Med 1996; 1:125–132.
5. Dietrich EB, Ndiayer M, Reed DM. Stenting in the carotid artery. Initial experience in 110 patients. J Endovasc Surg 1996; 3:42–62.
6. Theron J, Curtheoux P, Alachkar F, et al. A new triple catheter system for carotid angioplasty with cerebral protection. Am J Neuro Radiol 1990; 11(8):69–74.
7. Naylor AR, Bolia A, Abbot R, et al. Randomized study of carotid angioplasty and stenting versus carotid endarterectomy. A stopped trial. J Vasc Surg 1998; 28:326–334.
8. Gray-Weale AC. Carotid artery atheroma comparison of preoperative B mode ultrasound with carotid endarterectomy

specimens for pathology. J Cardiovasc Surg 1988; 29:676–681.

9. Lusby RJ, Ferrell LD, Ahrenfield WK, et al. Carotid plaque haemorrhage. Its role in the production of cerebral ischaemia. Arch Surg 1982; 117:1479–1488.

10. Gaunt ME, Ratliffe DA, Martin PJ, et al. On table diagnosis of incipient carotid artery thrombosis during carotid endarterectomy by transcranial doppler scanning. J Vasc Surg 1994; 20:104–107.

11. Matthias K. Katheterbehandlung der arteriellen voschlis skarankheit supraaortber gefasse. Radiologe 1987; 27:547–554.

12. Major ongoing stroke trials. Carotid and vertebral artery transluminal angioplasty study (CAVATAS). Stroke 1996; 27:358.

13. Begg C, Cho M, Eastwood S, et al. Improving the quality of reporting of randomised controlled trials. The Consort Statement. JAMA 1996; 276:637–639.

14. REM J. Interventional Radiol 1998; Suppl 9:162–166.

5
Angioplasty and Stenting at the Carotid Bifurcation, Part II

Patrice Frank Bergeron, Paul André Pietri, Patrick G. Khanoyan, and Vincent Maurice Louis Piret
Foundation Hospital Saint Joseph, Marseilles, France

Angioplasty and stenting has for a long time been limited to specific lesions of the internal or common carotid arteries, while surgery was the preferred treatment for carotid bifurcation. We believe that carotid bifurcation angioplasty and stenting (CBAS) has a limited role, which must be clearly defined. As vascular surgeons involved since 1990 in carotid angioplasty for selected lesions, we expect that this new way of treatment will resolve some critical situations either due to the type of lesion or to the patient itself but that it will not replace carotid surgery.

From the first carotid endarterectomy (CEA) performed by Eastcott and Rob in 1954, carotid surgery did has evolved, improving its technique and clarifying its indications. Surgery proved superior to medical treatment only after the large randomized trials performed in the 1990s (1–3). These trials proved justification of CEA in stroke prevention for stenosis more than 50%.

Percutaneous transluminal angioplasty (PTA) and stenting, thanks to brain protective devices, promise to improve results. Even if carotid stenting technique is evolving and will get better, opponents to this new technique cannot take advantage of its imperfections, if its use is restricted to patients who are high surgical risks. PTA is a useful adjuctive therapy in our arsenal. Without comparative randomized trials we cannot adequately compare these two techniques.

I. TECHNIQUES

This is an important point to standardize to allow all physicians involved in carotid therapy, such as vascular surgeons, to perform these new techniques. We believe that surgeons must be trained in carotid access either by the femoral route or by the simpler cervical approach. Several aspects and limitations should be considered to select the route of vascular access. The techniques of femoral or cervical access to carotid stenting have been previously de-scribed (4,5), so only some specific points will be discussed here concerning their indications, advantages, and disadvantages. Carotid catheterization via the femoral approach is one of the most difficult to perform and needs training and experience. The cervical approach is simpler but needs specific precautions including small-size introducers (5 or 6 F) and low dose of heparin (2000 IU). Antiplatelet drugs are given only the day before stenting, and the use of sealing devices with a plug outside the vessel is advantageous.

A. Advantages and Disadvantages of Cervical Access

Direct carotid puncture is often used after failure of the femoral approach (5% of cases). It is a simple and quick procedure that also can be done through a short skin incision 2 cm above the clavicle if the patient is anticoagulated. This approach avoids intra-aortic arch manipulations, which can be a source of brain embolisation.

The main disadvantage is discomfort for the patient and the physician when the procedure is performed under local anesthesia. We advise, if there is no contraindication, use at a light general anesthesia. In this case the intracranial flow should be monitored with a transcranial doppler (TCD) to record the middle cerebral artery circulation and detect any embolization.

B. Advantages and Disadvantages of Femoral Access

Femoral access is routine for diagnostic catheterization and allows treatment of all the vessels involved in the cerebral circulation. A femoral retrograde procedure is easy when the iliac flow is normal. This access allows periprocedural anticoagulation as is used for coronary angioplasty. One of the main advantages is the neurological monitoring that is possible with local anesthesia.

One disadvantage is the length of the devices needed, which can be a source of friction for nonflexible stents and associated with a lack of pushability. This approach requires training and has a learning curve. The main disadvantage is the potential risk of brain embolization during arch catheterization mainly when the arch or its branches are tortuous or diseased.

C. Selection of Access

To decide which access will be selected we examine aortic arch angiography and a CT scan. Two situations occur, depending on the anatomy and pathology of the arch. A normal arch curvature without arterial disease allows a quick, easy, safe procedure by a femoral approach. This should be the preferred choice allowing local anesthesia and perma-

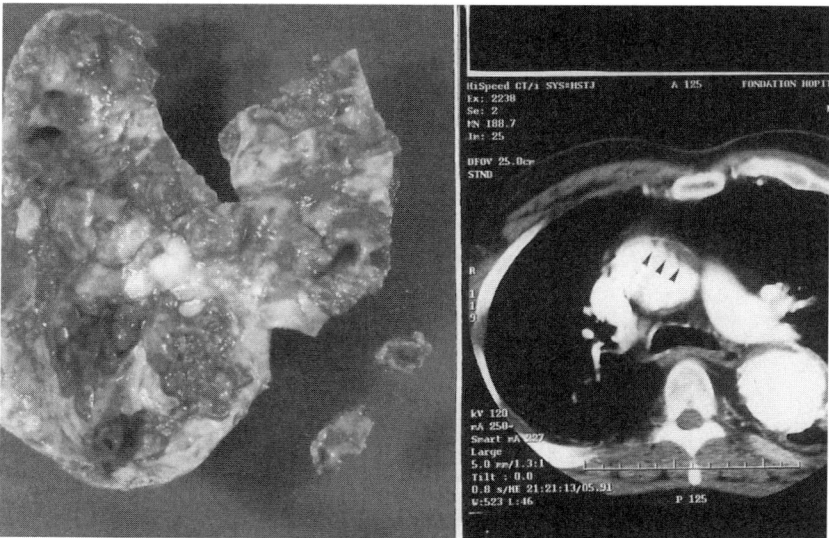

Figure 1 Gross morphology and CT scan of a diseased aortic arch. Note that the thrombi are clearly seen on the CT (arrowheads).

nent neurological control. In our practice, about 70% of patients are now treated by this means. When the aortic arch is diseased (Fig. 1) or if the course of the catheter is expected to be complex (Fig. 2), manipulations during the catheterization may be at high embolic risk. Similar tortuosities or anomalies of the common carotid artery (CCA) also prompt us to choose carotid access (Fig. 3). About 30% of our accesses are by direct cervical puncture. We have no experience with brachial access.

To avoid discomfort for the patient, carotid access is conducted under general anesthesia (if here is no contraindication). However, it can be done under local anesthesia. The lack of permanent neurological control is not more detrimental than it is for carotid surgery and the superiority of local anesthesia in terms of neurological complications has not been proven. The main element is to detect during the procedure any brain emboli. This is the role of TCD and

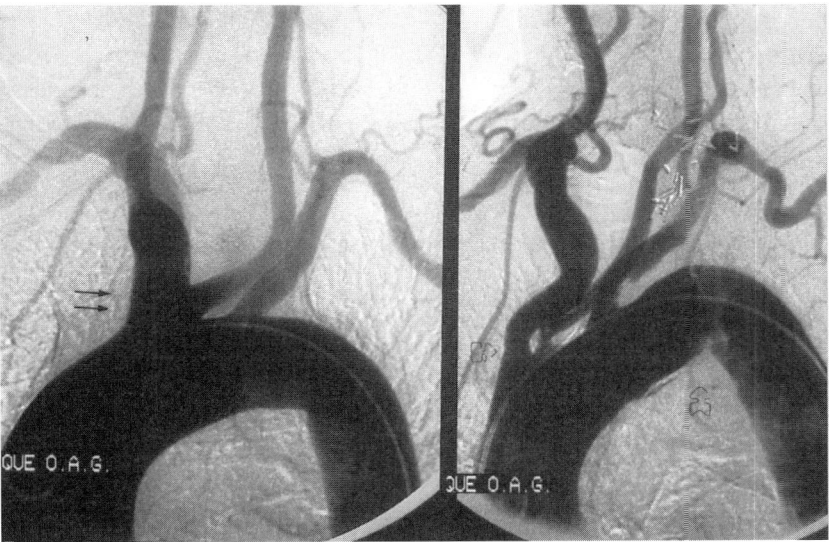

Figure 2 Two examples of complex arch anatomy for carotid catheterization.

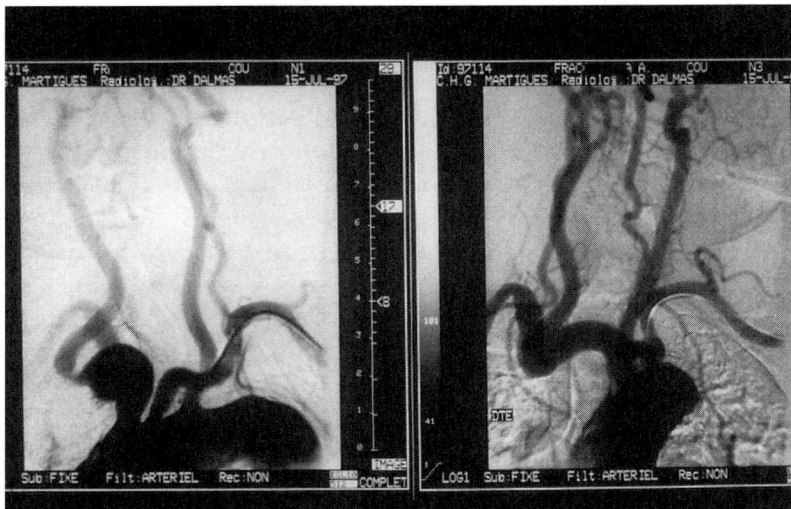

Figure 3 Complex tortuosity of the supra-aortic vessels predictive of a difficult catheterization of the common carotid artery.

intracranial angiography to look for any emboli or arterial interruption that would necessitate a specific neurorescue maneuver such as catheter thromboaspiration or thrombolysis.

II. CLINICAL EXPERIENCE AND RESULTS

Our total experience of 212 cases is described in Table 1. We started percutaneous carotid angioplasty without stenting in 1989, for fibromuscular dysplasia and some distal recurrent stenosis in the internal carotid artery (ICA). From 1990 to 1993, our experience was limited to 19 non-atherosclerotic diseased ICAs with selected stents for dissection after balloon angioplasty (BA) or residual stenosis. Our first stent was a half Palmaz-Schatz stent for recoil after balloon angioplasty of a recurrent stenosis in 1991. The experience of balloon angioplasty alone was inter-

Table 1   Clinical Personal Experience 1990–1999

	Balloon dilatation	Stenting	Total
Innominate artery	3	3	6
Common carotid artery (CCA)	3	18	21
Carotid bifurcation[a] (CB)	3	15	18
Internal carotid artery (ICA)	17	97	114
Carotid aneurysms[b]	—	5	5
Vertebral arteries	7	2	9
Subclavian arteries[c]	14	23	37
External carotid artery (ECA)	2	—	2
	49	163	212

[a] Almost all carotid bifurcation stenoses have been operated on.
[b] Carotid aneurysms have been treated by covered stents.
[c] All subclavian arteries were associated with symptoms.

rupted in 1993 because of a high rate of neurocomplications including an 8% ipsilateral stroke or death rate.

From 1993 to 1998, we treated 119 lesions involving the ICA in 77.5%, the CCA in 12%, and rarely the carotid bifurcation (CB) (7.5%). The techniques consisted of nonprotected direct stenting without predilatation in 93% of cases and the results were much better with a 1.7% stroke death/rate and 2.5% incidence of transient ischemic attacks (TIAs). There were no myocardial infarctions.

From January 1999 to October 1999, 23 patients were treated using a protective device (Percusurge). The selection of patients was modified by the use of this protective device, with an increased number of CB from 7.5% to 31.5% (Table 2). No ipsilateral complications occurred. One patient had a contralateral fatal stroke. This patient presented a common origin of the left and right CCA; an excessive flush in the right carotid artery sent debris to the left side.

Table 3 shows the immediate and late complications of our total personal experience and Table 4 shows the ipsilateral stroke and death rate in the different periods.

Table 2 Change in the Enrollment of Patients with the Use of a Protective Device

	Before January 1999 (no protection)	After January 1999 (routine protective device)
CCA	15%	15.8%
ICA	77.5%	52.6%
C. bifurcation	7.5%	31.5%

Table 3 Global Results of the Carotid Stenting Procedures

Immediate results		
1 Cervical asymptomatic AV fistula	0.7%
3 Technical failure	2.3%
3 Conversions	2.3%
2 Thrombosis	1.5%
4 TIA	3%
1 Minor stroke	0.7%
2 Major stroke ⇒ 2 death	1.5% (1 contralateral)
0 Myocardial infarction	0%

Late results: mean FU 27 months (1–98)

1 Conversion	0.7% (out-stent disease)
3 Stent compression	2.3%
4 Restenosis	3.1%
Stent patency	97.7% (1 late occlusion)

Stroke freedom 99% (1 non-stent-related TIA) and (1 symptomatic Palmaz stent compression)

Table 4 Evolution of the Ipsilateral Stroke Death Rate According to the Technique Used

1990–1993:	19 BA + selected stenting	8%
1993–1998:	119 Direct stenting	1.7%
1999:	23 Protected stenting (1 contralateral fatal stroke)	0%

Long-term results are satisfactory. The mean follow-up is 27 months (1–98). All patients were followed by duplex scan. Angiography was performed in some cases. Eight patients died in the follow-up period; none of the deaths were stent related. The stroke freedom was 99%. One patient had a TIA after a Palmaz stent traumatic compression, and one other had a non-stent-related TIA.

III. DISCUSSION AND PERSONAL OPINION REGARDING TECHNIQUES AND INDICATIONS

1. The feasibility of carotid stenting has been clearly demonstrated by previous series (6–9).

2. The safety of this approach has not been demonstrated by a comparison with surgery, with regard to carotid bifurcation. Nevertheless different series have reported a combined stroke/death rate of less than 10% and less than 5% when a direct stenting technique was used (6–9). The best results have been published by Theron using his own cerebral protective device (10,11). Some recent reports (M. Henry, personal communication, 1999) and our personal experience with the Percusurge device are encouraging and seems to minimize direct embolic complications. There is no doubt in our opinion that protective devices are effective and they should be mandatory during any angioplasty whatever the etiology of the lesion. From our experience, in all lesions we have collected debris from the site of angioplasty (Fig. 4). The amount of debris is greater for atherosclerotic lesions but debris is also released with stenting of recurrent stenoses, in stent restenoses, and carotid aneurysms. In our previous experience and that of others, without protection minor embolizations have been ignored because of the small size of the debris or because the cerebral infarction was in a silent area. This is commonly called "stroke of luck" but it is not a scientific, re-

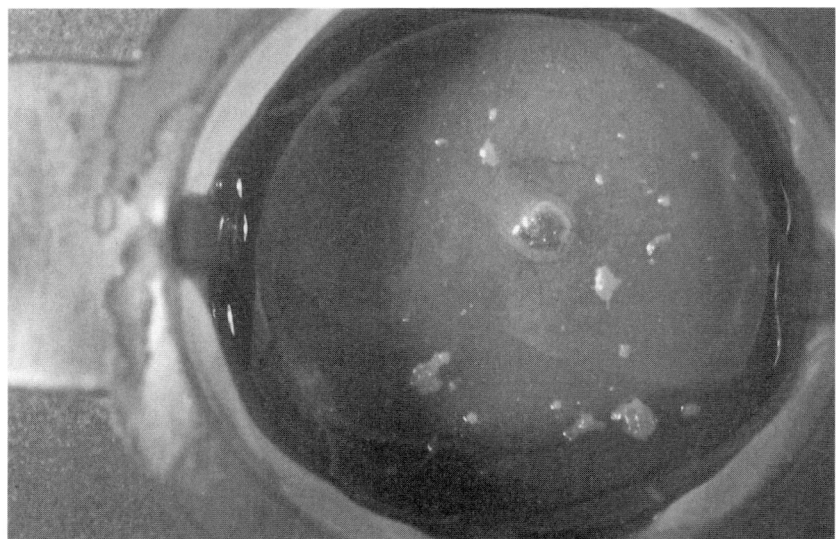

Figure 4 Debris collected by aspiration after protected carotid angioplasty.

sponsible approach. Carotid angioplasty should be considered a technique that carries a high risk of embolization. Thus, protection is of primary importance for neuronal preservation.

Other devices have been proposed for brain protection. Filters have been used by others (Roubin and Yadav, personal communications, 1999) and an occlusive balloon of the CCA with flow inversion (arteria) has been proposed by Parodi (personal communication, 1999).

3. Stents remain a great challenge at the level of the bifurcation. If we look at the CCA or ICA, this straight carotid segment can be recanalized in a satisfactory way in terms of the resulting image and flow; the plaque is remodeled and the stenosis is cured. At this level all stents are effective, some are balloon or self-expandable, their radial force is different, and their flexibility is an important feature. For a long time, our preference has been the Palmaz

stent because of its precise placement, its strong radial strength, and excellent long-term patency with a very low restenosis rate of 3.1%. In our experience, the limitation of this stent is related to its crushability. We found that this occurs in only 2.3% of patients if short stents, 2 cm or less, are used. The wall stent was our second option because of its flexibility. Nevertheless it has reduced radial strength and it is difficult to place precisely. The Nitinol stents such as those developed by Cordis or Guidant combine flexibility, high radial strength, and good deployment precision. These stents are new and we are not yet aware of their long-term results or their instent restenosis rates.

What about stenting the carotid bifurcation? The problem is more complex and there is no satisfactory bifurcated stent. Dealing with this problem one should choose between covering the external ostium (Fig. 5) or using beveled stents. Coverage of the external carotid artery (ECA) has been advocated as the ECA can usefully be occluded without complications. We believe that this artery has to be protected as a source of blood supply to the vertebrobasilar circulation. Moreover, neurological complications related to the ECA has been reported and we have experience with one patient presenting TIAs originating from an occluded ECA (Fig. 6). Remodeling of the bifurcation by angioplasty cannot be compared with a surgical repair. Surgery allows a perfect restoration of the carotid bifurcation. However, in some circumstances, such as with high-risk patients, we can accept covering the ECA for the value of restoring the IC lumen. What industry calls a carotid stent is a tapered stent, laser cut in a Nitinol tube with the small end in the ICA and the large end in the CCA. The placement precision of these self-expandable stents has been greatly enhanced. We have developed the concept of a beveled tubular stent to be placed in bifurcations (Fig. 7).

In-stent restenosis seems relatively slow and uncommon, occurring in less than 5% of cases in all published series. However, there is no doubt that the length of the

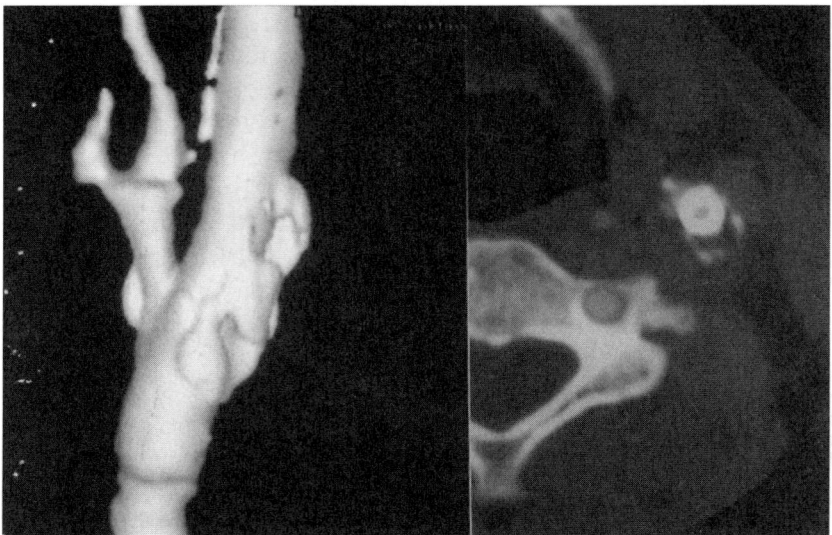

Figure 5 Three-dimensional CT scan example of a wall stent across the bifurcation, from the ICA to the CCA, covering the ECA ostium. Note in the right view that the stent is not applied to the arterial wall.

stent, its biocompatibility, and permanent wall stress are a source of myointimal hyperplasia. The shortest stent is the best. Nevertheless, asymptomatic in-stent restenosis does not need correction because of the low risk of embolization.

Is there a place for covered stents? No study can today answer this question except for carotid aneurysms, where they are mandatory.

4. How to manage a poorly tolerated occlusion of the ICA? Filters will probably solve this problem because of the carotid flow preservation. When an occlusive balloon is used, the procedure must be achieved very quickly. This can be done, according to our experience, in 4 min with the Percusurge device. This is an acceptable occlusive time. If the procedure is undertaken with general anesthesia, no

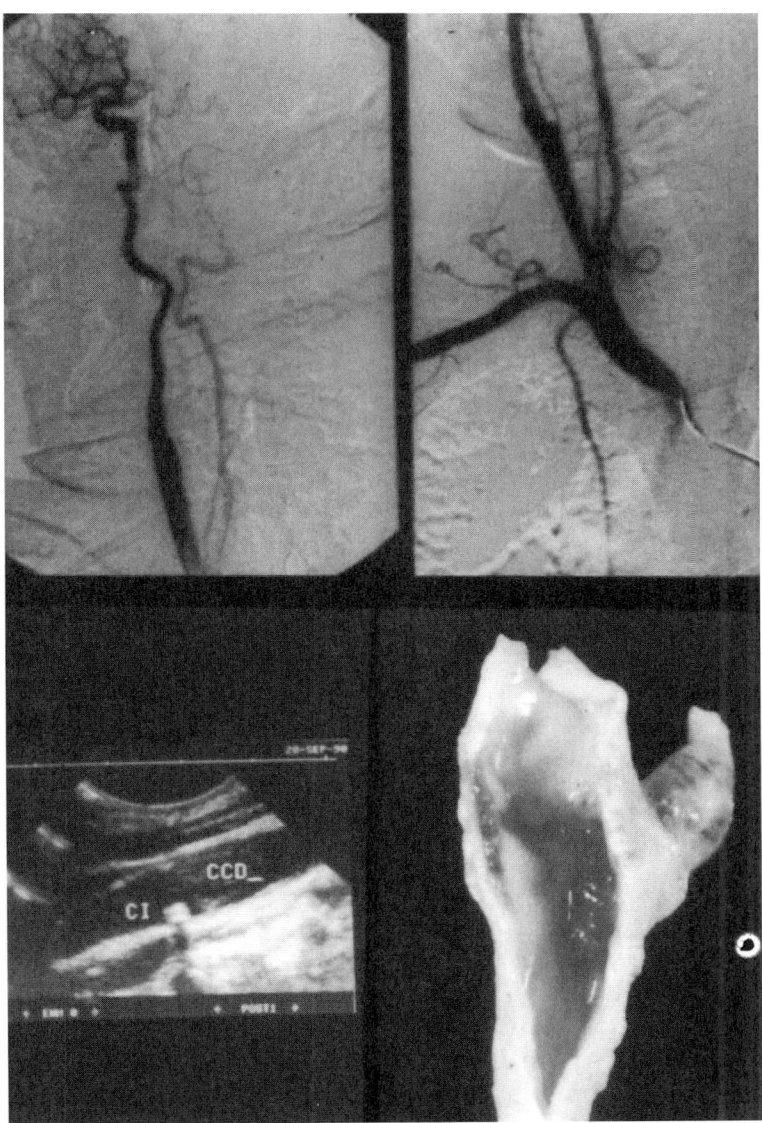

Figure 6 Example of a case of symptomatic external carotic artery occlusion. (Left and right top) Occlusion of the right ECA. (Left bottom) Duplex scan showing thrombus originating from the ECA. (Right bottom) View of the specimen removed at surgery. Note the thrombus in the occluded ECA sending clot debris to the ICA.

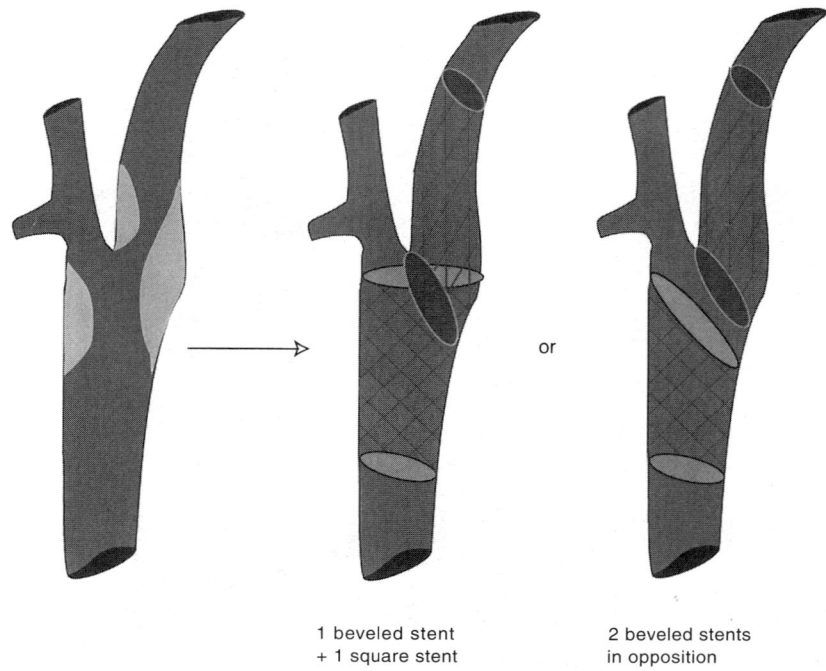

1 beveled stent   2 beveled stents
+ 1 square stent   in opposition

Figure 7 Carotid bifurcation stenting with the use of beveled stents.

convulsions or seizure will occur and the patient may recover completely after flow restoration.

5. Cardiac risk during carotid stenting seems to be extremely reduced in the different published series, except for
some bradycardias that appear during dilation of the carotid bifurcation. In our experience we have not had a myocardial infarction (MI): We already favor carotid angioplasty
for patients presenting with unstable or severe angina who
are candidates for either coronary angioplasty or a bypass.
Carotid stenting can be performed either the day before
surgery or concomitant with coronary angioplasty.

A. Indications

The variety of patients and lesions need precise criteria for selection. Surgical indications are clear compared to those of carotid stenting. Specific data exist from isolated experiences, some registries (12), and a few multicenter randomized trials. CAVATAS is the only one published (13); CREST is about to start (14).

Surgery is beneficial for symptomatic patients presenting with carotid stenosis >50% and asymptomatic patients with stenosis >70%. Until now patients must not be treated by routine PTA since we lack comparative data. However, symptomatic patients or these who need to have a carotid repair (mainly for bilateral lesions) and who are at high risk for surgery should be considered for stenting. However, risk criteria need to be carefully defined in this regard. Indications depend on multiple factors:

> The morphological aspect of the lesion based on duplex scan analysis. Echolucent plaques are at high risk for embolization, and should probably be operated on.
> The topography of the lesion.

High distal ICA stenosis or proximal supra-aortic lesions can easily be treated by angioplasty and stenting. On the contrary, the carotid bifurcation is easily accessible for surgery and often very complex or calcified for angioplasty and stenting. In Figure 8, we propose a classification of suitable and nonsuitable location of disease for CBAS. Figure 9 shows a scheme for our favorite current choice between surgery and stenting depending on the level of the carotid disease.

> The patient's neurological status; those with residual stroke need to have the simplest technique of repair under local anesthesia.
> The risk for nerve damage in case of previous neck surgery or radiotherapy.

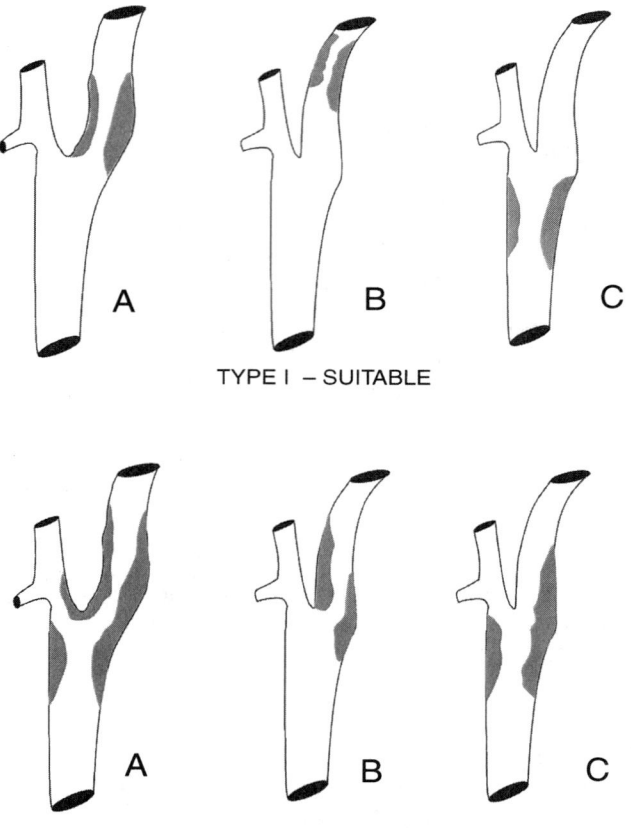

TYPE I – SUITABLE

TYPE I I – UNSUITABLE
(EXCEPT FOR HIGH RISK PATIENT OR HOSTILE NECKS)

Figure 8   Indication of carotid bifurcation angioplasty and stenting according to the topography of the lesion.

Patients with cardiac and pulmonary disease, mainly unstable angina, are more suitable for stenting, patients with complete circle of Willis or patients who will not tolerate carotid occlusion are preferably treated by stenting filters may be of greater use in this situation.

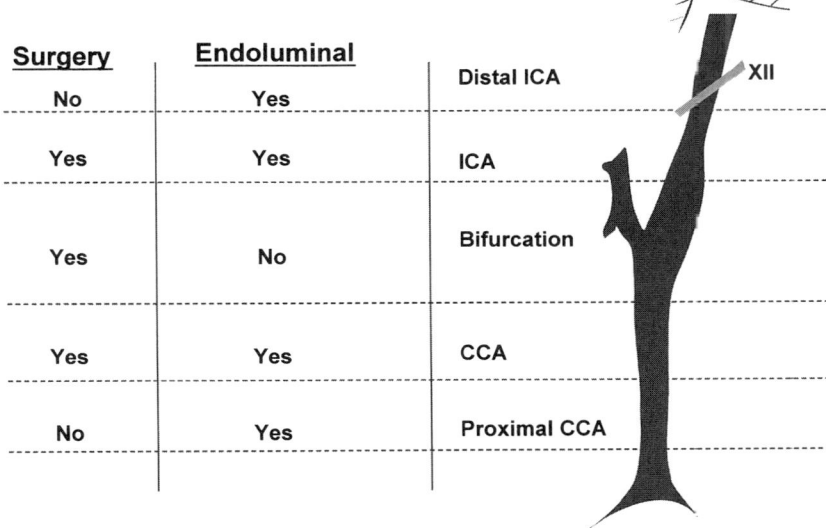

Surgery	Endoluminal	
No	Yes	Distal ICA
Yes	Yes	ICA
Yes	No	Bifurcation
Yes	Yes	CCA
No	Yes	Proximal CCA

Figure 9 Current optimal choice between surgery and endoluminal treatment according to the level of carotid disease.

Patients with coagulation disorders due to hepatic or bone marrow diseases, congenital or Iatrogenic, are not good candidates for surgery.
Patients under 65 or with long life expectancy need a proven technique such as surgery.

B. Contraindications to CBAs

These include patients who do not need carotid repair, patients at low risk, patients with a long life expectancy, patients with unsuitable lesions (extensive calcifications, ICA kinks or loops), patients with a suspected floating thrombus, acute thrombosis, and total occlusion, those with diffuse common carotid disease, string sign, recent stroke <2 weeks.

C. Indications for CBAs

These include patients with hostile necks, radiation, radical neck surgery, recurrent stenosis after CEA, frozen neck, and a high lesion, high-risk patients with indications for a carotid repair, those with overt cardiac disease (congestive heart failure, unstable angina), intracerebral flow impairment (contralateral occlusion, intracranial stenosis), short life expectancy (age or disease), multiple medical comorbidity.

IV. PREDICTIONS

We believe that carotid stenting will evolve with improved techniques and results. In the future we believe that embolic protection will be totally reliable and the immediate results of carotid stenting will compete favorably with surgery.

However, the long-term results, mainly the recurrence rate, are unknown, and this factor has to influence our current indications. If the long-term results at 5 years are comparable with surgery, the place of carotid stenting will increase and it will be used to treat most stenoses of the ICA, the CCA, and the origin of the supra-aortic trunks.

As for carotid bifurcation, stenting will be used for high-risk patients, mainly old patients with cardiac, respiratory, or neurological impairment. Young patients without specific risks will still be operated on to obtain a perfect anatomical result at the carotid bifurcation.

V. CONCLUSION

Carotid bifurcation angioplasty and stenting currently has limited specific indications. Long-term results and comparative studies mainly for high-risk patients are necessary before widening these indications. Surgery wil remain the gold standard for a majority of patients with carotid bifurcation disease.

REFERENCES

1. North American Symptomatic Carotid Endarterectomy Trial collaborators. Beneficial effect of carotid endarterectomy in symptomatic patients with high-grade carotid stenosis. N Engl J Med 1991; 325:445–453.
2. European Carotid Surgery Trialists' Collaborative Group, European Carotid Surgery Trial. Interim results for symptomatic patients with severe (70–99%) or with mild (0–29%) carotid stenosis. Lancet 1991; 337:1235–1243.
3. Moore WS, Barnet HJM, Beebe HG, et al. Guidelines for carotid endarterectomy, a multidisciplinary consensus statement from the Ad Hoc Committee, American Heart Association. Stroke 1995; 26:188–201.
4. Bergeron P. Techniques endoluminales de traitement des lésions carotidiennes. Encycl Med Chir Techniques chirurgicales—Chirurgie vasculaire, Fa 43-141. Paris: Elsevier, 1998, 8 pp.
5. Bergeron P, Alexandrescu V, Liang E, Amichot A, Khanoyan P. Primary carotid stenting via cervical approach. In Henry M, Amor M, Theron J, Roubin G, eds. Carotid Angioplasty and Stenting. Europa ed. 1998:169–179.
6. Dietrich EB, Ndiaye M, Reid DB. Stenting in the carotid artery: initial experience in 100 patients. J Endovasc Surg 1996; 3:42–62.
7. Yadav JS, Roubin GS, Iyer SS, et al. Elective stenting of the extracranial carotid arteries. Circulation 1997; 95:376–381.
8. Henry M, Amor M, Henry I, et al. Endovascular treatment of atherosclerotic internal carotid artery stenosis. J Endovasc Surg 1997; 4(suppl I):1–14.
9. Bergeron P, Becquemin JP, Jausseran JM, Biasi G, Cardon JM, Castellani L, Martinez R, Florani P, Kniemeyer P. Percutaneous stenting of the internal carotid artery: the European CAST I Study. J Endovasc Surg 1999; 6:155–159.

10. Theron J, Courtheoux P, Alachkar, et al. New triple coaxial catheter system for carotid angioplasty with cerebral protection. Am J Neuro Radiol 1990; 11:869–874.
11. Theron J. Protected stenting of atherosclerotic stenoses at the carotid bifurcation. Radioàlogy 1998; 209:473.
12. Wholey MH, Wholey M, Bergeron P, et al. Current global status of carotid artery stent placement. Cathet Cardiovasc Diagn 1998; 44:1–6.
13. Brow MM. Vascular surgical society of Great Britain and Ireland: results of the carotid and vertebral artery transluminal angioplasty study. Br J Surg 1999; 86:710–711.
14. Hobson RW II, Brott T, Ferguson R, Roubin G, Moore W, Kuntz R, Howard G, Ferguson J. CREST: Carotid Revacularization Endarterectomy versus Stent Trial. Cardiovasc Surg 1997; (5):457–458.

6

Cervical Carotid Atherosclerotic Stenosis

Two Distinct Conditions

J. J. Connors III
Inova Fairfax Hospital, Falls Church, Virginia

Cervical carotid atherosclerotic stenosis (CCAS) causes significant morbidity and mortality. Stroke is the greatest cause of health care expenditure and is perhaps the most feared of all medical conditions.

Use of a single inclusive term for all brachiocephalic atherosclerotic disease (including intracranial atherosclerotic stenosis) is imprecise for discussion of this group of conditions. Extensive research concerning CCAS has been performed. This has been motivated by the fact that CCAS is relatively easy to evaluate, not uncommon, a major health threat, and possibly correctable. CCAS is unique in vascular pathology in that the threat is of an embolic nature rather than hemodynamic. This is completely different from the threat posed by vascular disease in the heart, legs, or kidneys, for instance.

In a fashion similar to malignant versus benign neoplasms, there are two distinct types of cervical carotid atherosclerotic stenosis with two distinct sets of symptoms and prognoses: embologenic and nonembologenic. Embologenic CCAS is associated with recurrent episodes of neurological dysfunction (transient ischemic attacks, TIAs) whereas nonembologenic CCAS is asymptomatic. Embologenic CCAS is associated with approximately a 10–15% annual risk of major stroke versus about 1–2% for nonembologenic CCAS. Types of plaque have been determined to correlate with risk profiles (echogenic, calcified, etc.) and may be of prognostic value.

I. THERAPEUTIC OPTIONS

A. Medical Therapy

Prior dogma determined that medical therapy neither significantly affected the progression of atherosclerosis nor caused its regression. Certain environmental factors (tobacco, foods, etc.) specifically worsen atherosclerosis. Recent data indicate that particular pharmaceuticals can slow its progression (statins, antihomocysteine therapies, etc). Warfarin and aspirin have been shown to have no effect on atherosclerosis.

No trial has evaluated currently available "best medical therapy" for CCAS (which might include warfarin, ticlopidine, glycoprotein IIb-IIIa inhibitors, etc.). While antiplatelet medication (aspirin or aspirin/dipyridamole, etc.) has been shown to be effective for stroke reduction for embologenic brachiocephalic atherosclerotic disease, aspirin therapy is still associated with about 10–15% annual risk of stroke for embologenic CCAS. However, when CCAS has an asymptomatic history (i.e., is apparently the nonembologenic type) the risk of stroke is very low and antiplatelet therapy is not as urgently indicated and may be of minimal absolute benefit. Indeed, intervention of any kind (i.e., endarterectomy) is of debatable benefit for this condition.

The benefits of carotid endarterectomy in the setting of nonembologenic (asymptomatic) carotid artery disease are not well established. Four trials comparing medical therapy to endarterectomy for asymptomatic carotid stenosis have been completed (1–4). Three of these four showed no positive benefit for endarterectomy and all showed commensurately low rates of stroke with medical therapy alone. The Mayo Asymptomatic Carotid Endarterectomy Trial was prematurely terminated due to a significantly higher number of myocardial infarctions and transient ischemic events in the surgical group even though these were comparable to other surgical series.

Only the Asymptomatic Carotid Atherosclerosis Study (ACAS) demonstrated a benefit of endarterectomy for asymptomatic carotid stenosis. ACAS evaluated patients with stenoses of greater than 60% (1). The 5-year natural history risk of ipsilateral stroke was shown to be 11.0% (2.2% annual rate). The total 5-year risk of stroke was reduced by surgical endarterectomy to 5.1% (1.0% annual rate). This, however, was only a decrease of 1% per year, mostly accounted for by a reduction in minor strokes, not major strokes. The ECST Collaborative Group studied 2295 asymptomatic carotid stenoses ranging from 0% to 99% for an average of 4.5 years (5). The 3-year stroke risk in 127 patients with stenoses of 70–99% (50–99% by NASCET criteria) was 5.7% (1.9% annual rate). Another large series confirmed that the risk of moderate (50–79% by NASCET criteria) asymptomatic stenosis was very low (6). With life-table analysis the estimated cumulative risk of ipsilateral stroke was 0.85% in one year, 3.6% in 3 years, and 5.4% in 5 years (6). Additional studies have confirmed the low intrinsic risk of asymptomatic carotid stenosis (7–9). Most risk is associated with a stenosis greater than approximately 80%, corresponding to a residual lumen of approximately 1 mm or less (10).

These preliminary data imply that the major risk associated with CCAS disease is the presence of symptoms, not necessarily the degree of stenosis. For a symptomatic patient, a moderate stenosis appears to be a higher risk for ipsilateral stroke than a more severe stenosis in an asymptomatic patient (11–14).

As opposed to ACAS, which recommended carotid endarterectomy for asymptomatic patients with angiographically proven stenosis of more than 60%, the Canadian Stroke Consortium reached consensus that there was insufficient evidence to endorse this procedure for *any* level of asymptomatic stenosis (15). Reasons cited were lack of proof of reduction of the risk of major disabling stroke, the question of reproducibility of surgical results in the general population, and the unproven long-term benefit of surgical reconstruction. Because of a lack of convincing positive data, others have suggested further trials to evaluate the efficacy of endarterectomy for asymptomatic carotid artery stenosis (16).

Recently published data indicate a significantly higher perioperative death rate for unselected Medicare patients undergoing carotid endarterectomy at the same institutions participating in the NACSET and/or ACAS studies than for the original study patients (0.6% for NASCET patients, 0.1% for ACAS patients, but 1.4% for all Medicare patients) (17). The perioperative mortality rate for Medicare patients undergoing carotid endarterectomy at nonstudy sites was 1.7% for high-volume institutions, 1.9% for average-volume institutions, 2.5% for low-volume institutions when unselected Medicare patients were considered. The morbidity rate in these trials has routinely been several times that of mortality. The patients participating in the NASCET and ACAS trials were younger and healthier than the typical Medicare patients undergoing endarterectomy at the same or other institutions. These results of the unselected Medicare patients are particularly alarming considering that they are combined statistics from symptomatic and asymptomatic patients and realizing that asymptomatic patients should have a death rate of 0.1%. In addition, the severe stroke rate is generally thought to be several times the death rate, resulting in an estimated combined rate far higher than those reported in the trials.

B. Risk Management for CCAS

Certain types of stenosis (echogenic, calcific, etc.) have been shown to carry variable degrees of risk independent of degrees of stenosis. Embologenicity is a strong predictor of major stroke risk. Even utilizing optimal medical therapy, intervention for certain types of CCAS is necessary. Endarterectomy is a technique with proven efficacy and reasonably low morbidity and mortality for certain, carefully selected, patients. Specific patients pose higher surgical risks than others and may require an alternative therapy.

C. Nonmedical (Revascularization) Therapies

Endarterectomy

Aggressiveness of intervention for any medical condition depends on at least three broad areas of concern: 1) ongoing symptom severity and patient discomfort, 2) probability and severity of the eventual major threat, and 3) ease, safety, and effectiveness of the method of intervention. The degree of risk and patient discomfort (symptom) profiles for embologenic CCAS mandate effective therapy. There is ongoing debate regarding the need for aggressive intervention with nonembologenic (asymptomatic) CCAS.

Several trials have validated the effectiveness of carotid endarterectomy (CEA) for carefully selected patients with severe embologenic CCAS when performed by selected surgeons. Recent data indicate that the results of CEA as currently practiced do not match the North American Symptomatic Carotid Endarterectomy Trial (NASCET) or Asymptomatic Carotid Atherosclerosis Study (ACAS), and CEA may not be safer or more effective than currently available medical therapy for a large percentage of patients actually undergoing endarterectomy.

Carotid Stenting

There is a high level of interest in carotid stenting but a lack of definitive proof of safety, efficacy, or durability. The relatively good results attained with this procedure at certain institutions are commendable and encouraging; however, it must be appreciated that these results have generally been achieved by utilization of numerous physical resources and the involvement of skilled personnel from many disciplines. Until clinically validated, carotid artery angioplasty and stenting should be reserved for those patients at high risk for stroke, the best candidates being high-surgical-risk symptomatic patients with significant comorbidity. Carotid stenting under these circumstances may offer a less invasive means than endarterectomy for favorably influencing the risk of stroke and can be viewed as "acceptable, but not yet proven."

Carotid stenting with embolic control may offer a low-risk alternative for high-surgical-risk patients. Indeed, with an effective means of embolic control, carotid stenting is intrinsically a lower physical stress procedure than surgery for the patient.

II. CONCLUSIONS

There is incomplete knowledge concerning CCAS disease, its specific risk characteristics, current optimal medical therapy, indications for intervention, and the optimal means to do so. No trial has evaluated currently available "best medical therapy" for CCAS or compared this to endarterectomy. Current data indicate that carotid endarterectomy as it is currently practiced in the United States bears little relationship to the populations studied, methods used, or results obtained in the NASCET and ACAS studies. There is legitimate disagreement on the need for aggressive intervention for nonembologenic (asymptomatic) CCAS. There is a high level of interest in carotid stenting but a lack of definitive proof of safety, efficacy, or durability. Carotid stenting can be performed with a reasonable degree of safety. Until clinically validated, carotid stenting as presently performed should be reserved for patients at high risk for stroke.

Cerebral protection from procedural emboli during carotid stenting can potentially reduce the risk of carotid stenting to a level comparable to that of endarterectomy or even lower. Carotid stenting may therefore *potentially* offer an improved therapeutic strategy for risk management of CCAS. Further study is warranted.

REFERENCES

1. Asymptomatic Carotid Atherosclerosis Study Executive Committee. Endarterectomy for asymptomatic carotid artery stenosis. JAMA 1995; 273:1421–1428.
2. Hobson RW II, Weiss DG, Fields WS, et al. Efficacy of carotid endarterectomy for asymptomatic carotid stenosis. The Vet-

erans Affairs Cooperative Study Group. N Engl J Med 1993; 328:221–227.

3. The CASANOVA Study Group. Carotid surgery versus medical therapy in asymptomatic carotid stenosis. Stroke 1991; 22:1229–1235.

4. Mayo Asymptomatic Carotid Endarterectomy Study Group. Results of a randomized controlled trial of carotid endarterectomy for asymptomatic carotid stenosis. Mayo Clin Proc 1992; 67:513–518.

5. European Carotid Surgery Trialists Collaborative Group. Risk of stroke in the distribution of an asymptomatic carotid artery. Lancet 1995; 345:209–212.

6. Rockman CB, Riles TS, Lamparello PJ, Giangola G, Adelman MA. Natural history and management of the asymptomatic, moderately stenotic internal carotid artery. J Vasc Surg 1997; 25:423–431.

7. Hennerici M, Hulsbomer HB, Hefter H, Lammerts D, Rautenberg W. Natural history of symptomatic extracranial arterial disease. Results of a long term prospective study. Brain 1987; 110(part 3):777–791.

8. Olin JW, Fonseca C, Childs MB, et al. The natural history of asymptomatic moderate internal carotid artery stenosis by duplex ultrasound. Vasc Med 1998; 3:101–108.

9. Irvine CD, Cole SE, Foley PX. Unilateral asymptomatic carotid disease does not require surgery. Eur J Vasc Surg 1998; 16:245–253.

10. Chambers BR, Norris JW. Outcome in patients with asymptomatic neck bruits. N Engl J Med 1986; 315:860–865.

11. North American Symptomatic Carotid Endarterectomy Trial Collaborators. Beneficial effect of carotid endarterectomy in symptomatic patients with high-grade carotid stenosis. N Engl J Med 1991; 325:445–453.

12. Barnett HJ, Taylor DW, Eliasziw M, et al. Benefit of carotid endarterectomy in patients with symptomatic moderate or severe stenosis. N Engl J Med 1998; 339:1468–1471.

13. European Carotid Trialists Collaborative Group. MRC European Carotid Surgery Trial: interim results for symptomatic patients with severe (70% to 99%) or with mild (0 to 29%) carotid stenosis. Lancet 1991; 337:1235–1243.

14. European Carotid Surgery Trialists Collaborative Group.

Randomized trial of endarterectomy for recently symptomatic carotid stenosis: final results of the MRC European Carotid Surgery Trial (ECST). Lancet 1998; 351:1379–1387.

15. Perry JR, Szalai JP, Norris JW. Consensus against both endarterectomy and routine screening for asymptomatic carotid artery stenosis. Canadian Stroke Consortium. Arch Neurol 1996; 54:25–28.

16. Chaturvedi S, Halliday A. Is another clinical trial warranted regarding endarterectomy for asymptomatic carotid stenosis? Cerebrovasc Dis 1998; 8:210–213.

17. Wennberg DE, Lucas FL, Birkmeyer JD, Bredenberg CE, Fisher ES. Variation in carotid endarterectomy mortality in the Medicare population: trial hospitals, volume, and patient characteristics. JAMA 1998; 279:1278–1281.

7
The State of the Art of Carotid Bifurcation Angioplasty and Stenting

Edward B. Diethrich
Arizona Heart Institute and Arizona Heart Hospital, Phoenix, Arizona

I. INTRODUCTION

Although stents are not yet approved for use in the carotid artery, a number of investigators have published the results of early clinical studies. Endovascular treatment of lesions in the common carotid, bifurcation, and internal carotid arteries has been reported by a number of investigators (1–13). Results have been mixed but indicate that improvements in device design and delivery techniques may reduce complications. Indeed, technological advances in endovascular equipment have changed treatment strategies for vascular disease considerably over the last 10 years.

The subject of carotid bifurcation angioplasty and stenting remains highly controversial. To some extent, our work at the Arizona Heart Institute—which led to an early publication (6) on the subject of carotid stenting—may have fueled some of the initial debate. Although our initial unfavorable results were published in 1996, they continue to be cited in current reviews (14). It is certainly clear that we now need to establish rigid and consistent reporting standards that move us away from anecdotal experience with these procedures. The Food and Drug Administration (FDA), for instance, has stated unequivocally that carotid stenting is a procedure that should be performed only in centers that have obtained Institutional Review Board (IRB) approval and have an investigational device exemption (IDE). Clearly, this directive is being violated on a daily basis at a number of institutions around the country.

Although Hobson and colleagues have designed the CREST Trial (Carotid Revascularization Endarterectomy Versus Stent Trial) (15), our group and others contend that it may well be unethical to subject patients to a randomization scheme that directs them toward the classic surgical procedure when there are certain subgroups of patients (e.g., those who have been treated with radiation and radical neck dissection) in whom it is already clear that angioplasty and stenting is preferable to endarterectomy. The argument is well articulated by Wholey (16), who points out that proposed trials incorporate NASCET entry criteria despite the fact that most interventionists are stenting patients who are not NASCET eligible. He maintains that most surgeons would agree to initiate trials that include patients in high-risk surgical and medical groups and that this might be best done first in a registry. In addition, he discusses the problems of establishing a large trial. At present just 10–15 centers in the United States are responsible for 65% of all carotid stenting procedures, whereas an effective trial will require 40 clinical sites with trained interventionists. In addition, there is no ideal, dedicated delivery system for use in carotid stenting procedures and, apparently, a stent that has very limited application in the carotid has been selected for use in the CREST trial. Wholey suggests that trials should focus first on high-risk patients, and then proceed to the NASCET subset. Clearly, a great deal of study will be required to bring new procedures and devices for carotid intervention into safe and effective use.

II. RECENT EXPERIENCE WITH ANGIOPLASTY AND STENTING AT THE CAROTID BIFURCATION

Experience with endovascular intervention at the carotid bifurcation is still in the early stages, and the literature reviewing endovascular intervention at the carotid bifurcation is relatively scant at present. The potential for neurological complications is high at the bifurcation given the risk of embolic events from traversal of the lesion with an angioplasty catheter and balloon. Nevertheless, in certain subgroups of patients these techniques appear superior to carotid endarterectomy. In this setting, the endovascular procedure may be an appealing option, and we find ourselves in the position of comparing the results of endovascular intervention with those of endarterectomy.

Recent study in 105 patients (11) who underwent treatment of 115 carotid bifurcation stenoses (40 by angioplasty and stenting; 75 by carotid endarterectomy) indicates that levels of microemboli are higher in patients undergoing the endovascular procedure. In this retrospective study, transcranial Doppler monitoring detected a mean of 74.0 emboli per stenosis during endovascular treatment as compared to 8.8 emboli per stenosis during carotid endarterectomy ($p = 0.0001$). The postprocedural neurological events in the stenting group included two strokes (5.6%) and two transient ischemic attacks (5.6%). One patient (1.4%) who underwent endarterectomy had a stroke. Although these results indicate that the levels of emboli are higher during endovascular procedures, it remains to be seen whether these correlate with higher risk of morbidity and mortality in large, controlled trials. Additionally, it must be noted that this study, like so many others at present, incorporates the early learning curve of the investigational team.

In a recent comparison of stenting versus endarterectomy in carotid artery disease, 273 patients underwent treatment of 310 carotid bifurcation stenoses—107 were treated with stents, and 166 had an endarterectomy procedure (12). Major neurological complications were seen in six stented patients (5.6%) and in two endarterectomy patients (1.2%). At 6 months, follow-up was available in 193 patients (Table 1). The authors concluded that early results

Table 1 Comparison of Outcome with Stenting Versus Endarterectomy in the Carotid Bifurcation at 6-Month Follow-Up ($n = 193$)

Outcome	Stent therapy	Endarterectomy
Minor stroke	7 (6.5%)	1 (0.6%)
Major stroke	1 (0.9%)	1 (0.6%)
Death	4 (3.7%)	6 (3.6%)

Source: Ref. 12.

with stenting in this location were promising, but that the technique is not necessarily safer than endarterectomy. Still, the data suggest that stenting may be an alternative for the treatment of carotid artery bifurcation lesions in selected patients who are deemed to be at risk for complications associated with classic surgical intervention.

A cost comparison by the same group of investigators reviewed the clinical results and hospital charges in patients who underwent elective treatment for carotid stenosis (13). In this study, 218 patients were admitted a total of 229 times for 234 procedures to treat 239 carotid bifurcation stenoses (109 angioplasty and stenting; 130 carotid endarterectomy). The incidence of postprocedural strokes was 7.7% ($n = 8$) in the stent group and 1.5% ($n = 2$) in the endarterectomy group. There was one death in the stent group, and there were two deaths in the endarterectomy group. Although the length of stay was similar between groups (2.9 days in the stent group vs. 3.1 days in the endarterectomy group), total costs associated with hospital stay were $30,140 in the stent group and $21,670 in the endarterectomy group—the costs of equipment and imaging were greater and contributed to higher costs in the stent group. The authors concluded that stenting for carotid bifurcation stenoses cannot be justified on the basis of cost. Nevertheless, there may be other considerations that influence the choice of procedure, and we have certainly seen in other early investigations that the cost of devices and procedures declines as operator experience and competition among vendors supplying the equipment increases.

III. TECHNIQUES FOR CAROTID ARTERY ANGIOPLASTY AND STENTING

A. Anesthesia

Most endovascular procedures do not require the use of a general anesthetic. We prefer a local anesthesia with mild sedation for percutaneous retrograde femoral interventions. Agents that allow the patient to be completely comfortable and conversant during the procedure are preferred so that immediate assessment of any neurological change may be made (17–19). Neurological deficits from ischemia caused by balloon inflations are rare; rapid deflation quickly reverses the symptoms. Balloon inflation at the carotid bifurcation more commonly yields baroreceptor stimulation, causing bradycardia. Cardiac standstill may result, and momentary sternal compression may be required. One milligram of atropine sulfate administered 60 sec before balloon expansion usually prevents this complication but does not guarantee against it; careful attention should be paid to the ECG monitor during ballooning.

Short-acting, rapidly reversible drugs should be used when direct-access techniques are used, so the patient may be awake and extubated in the endovascular suite immediately following the procedure (17). Although cervical block and local anesthesia have been used successfully in carotid interventions (18,19), immobilizing the head and neck during the procedure is difficult, particularly if the patient is not intubated and the anesthesiologist must support a mask over the patient's face. Patient movement at the time of stent deployment increases the risk of incorrect placement of the device.

B. Access

The carotid region is usually accessed using a retrograde femoral approach, although direct common carotid artery access may also be indicated. In nearly all carotid procedures, a radiopaque ruler (Burkhart Roentgen, Pinellas Park, FL) is placed beneath the patient's shoulder and its position relative to the target carotid artery is confirmed with fluoroscopy. Since the lesions to be treated require imaging within the thorax, the fluoroscopic unit is moved over to the field, and radiopaque objects such as tubing and ECG leads are positioned so as not to interfere with imaging during the procedure.

Carotid Artery Access

Direct, percutaneous carotid access is associated with a relatively high rate of complications, and we no longer use it at our institution. Our current procedure employs a short, 2–3-cm incision just above the clavicle to expose the artery before insertion of the 18G needle. The common carotid artery is dissected free from the carotid sheath and held with a heavy silk or vessel loop. This variation in our technique avoids the potential for postprocedural hematoma and prevents stent compression seen with the percutaneous approach.

The techniques for antegrade and retrograde carotid artery access are identical except for their direction. The antegrade approach to the internal carotid artery is documented below.

The entry site into the common carotid artery can be variable distances above the clavicle, depending on the location of the lesion. A short incision (as described above) is made to expose a segment of the common carotid artery, and an 18G, 2 3/8-in. single-wall entry needle (Cook, Inc., Bloomington, IN) is used for the puncture. Several companies are now working on embolic protection devices. One of the devices we have been using is the PercuSurge guidewire system. This particular device incorporates a distal occluding balloon with the capacity for an irrigation system that aspirates debris created by balloon dilatation. Early results have been encouraging, but this method and others are still in the initial development stages.

In most cases, an angled hydrophilic guidewire such as the Glidewire (Meditech/Boston Scientific, Watertown, MA) is passed cephalad into the external carotid artery and crossing of the internal carotid artery is avoided as it may result in embolic complications. We use a 7F Coons dilator (Cook, Inc., Bloomington, IN) to expedite the sheath placement and then insert a 7F, 6-cm-long sheath (Cordis, Warren, NJ), releasing a short bolus of contrast to confirm sheath placement. A fluoroscopic road-mapping image is acquired on disk, and the fluoroscopic unit remains stationary for the rest of the procedure. Intravenous heparin sodium (approximately 5000 units) is given to maintain the activated coagulation time (ACT) above 250 sec, and the sheaths and catheters are irrigated with a heparinized saline solution (10,000 units of heparin to 1000 mL normal saline).

Although preprocedural duplex scanning is extremely valuable in assessing the nature of the lesion and the degree of narrowing, angiographic visualization is used to judge the length and diameter of the lesion and is the basis for deciding whether or not to predilate. Predilation is frequently necessary before stent deployment in severely stenotic lesions. Balloon diameter is usually one or two sizes smaller than the stent delivery balloon. Preparing the stent delivery balloon at this time shortens the interval between balloon predilation and stent deployment.

Selecting the appropriate stent depends upon the diameter and length of the lesion. The most common balloon dilation catheter size is a 4-mm-×-2-cm balloon followed by stent delivery on the same size or next-larger-sized balloon. In general, two types of stents are being used today, neither of which has been approved by the FDA for use in the carotid location. Several newer designs are under development, and corporate sponsors are initiating clinical trials of them. Most experience with stents to date has been gained using the rigid, balloon-expandable Palmaz stent (Cordis, Warren, NJ) or the Wallstent (Boston Scientific), which is a flexible, self-expanding stent.

After preparation of the balloon and stent, the guidewire is withdrawn from the external carotid artery, and a smaller Roadrunner wire (Cook, Inc., Bloomington, IN) is passed across the lesion into the internal carotid artery. The wire is kept low in the extracranial internal carotid artery to avoid any vascular trauma or arterial spasm. The anesthesiologist administers atropine (1 mg) to block bradycardia and resulting hypotension during balloon expansion.

The road-mapping image is used to help center the balloon across the lesion, and a short burst of contrast is injected to allow visualization of its final position. The balloon is expanded for a few seconds at 8–10 atmospheres. If bradycardia occurs, the balloon should be deflated immediately. When the expansion is complete and the balloon has been deflated, the shaft of the angioplasty catheter is rotated to furl the balloon before it is retracted. Contrast injection confirms the result of the balloon dilation and the establishment of an adequate passageway for stent deployment.

The balloon catheter with the stent is then advanced into position, and the stent is situated between the dots on the balloon. If the patient moves, and the road map is lost, a repeat contrast injection is necessary. When a rigid stent moves on the balloon or is misaligned, it should be repositioned—even if it requires complete removal of the balloon and stent delivery catheter. After the operator is satisfied with the stent's position, the balloon is expanded to deploy the device or, in the case of a self-expandable stent, the stent is simply released. A short inflation over 5 sec is generally sufficient for balloon expansion. The electrocardiogram should be carefully monitored for any changes.

Following stent deployment, contrast is injected to confirm patency and assess proper positioning. In all cases, regardless of the approach, a complete cerebral angiogram is performed at the conclusion of the stent deployment. This is particularly important to confirm the absence of cerebral embolization—a scenario requiring a neurorescue technique such as thrombolytic infusion. While it has not been our standard practice to image the intracranial area prior to manipulations across the carotid lesion, it might be advantageous to image at baseline for comparison with the control study. It has become clear that inadequate stent expansion contributes to complications such as stent occlusion and thrombus formation, and we frequently use real-time intravascular ultrasound to determine the adequacy of stent deployment.

Once the procedure is complete and the incision is closed, anesthesia may be discontinued. It is still important that blood pressure be monitored closely at this time as uncontrolled hypertension may result in significant hematoma formation. Before transfer, the patient should be awakened and assessed for any neurological deficits. After the transfer, we perform a duplex scan of the treatment site within the first hour.

Femoral Access

The retrograde femoral access method is the most familiar and frequently used access technique in endovascular intervention and is often used for both diagnostic and therapeutic modalities. Both iliac arteries are evaluated, and the side with the less tortuous and stenotic artery is chosen to facilitate the placement of the sheath and advancement of the guiding catheter into the aortic arch. Occlusion of abdominal aorta or the femoral/iliac vessels precludes retrograde femoral access; however, either a direct carotid or a brachial approach can be used.

An 18G, 2 3/8-in. needle is inserted in the common femoral artery and followed by a 0.035-in. guidewire (Glidewire, Medi-tech/Boston Scientific, Watertown, MA) and a 7F or 9F sheath (Cordis, Warren, NJ). Intravenous heparin (approximately 5000 units) is then administered, and a 260-cm, 0.035-in. angled hydrophilic guidewire (Medi-tech) is passed into the aortic arch. A JB2 catheter (Cook, Inc., Bloomington, IN) is passed into the high ascending aorta, and the wire is withdrawn to expose the angle of the JB2 catheter. The catheter is then pulled back slowly to selectively engage either the brachiocephalic trunk or the origin of the left common carotid artery. Once the angled guidewire has been passed into the appropriate common carotid artery, the JB2 catheter is advanced over it to the midlevel of the carotid artery. The angled guidewire is then passed into the external carotid artery followed by the JB2 catheter. The guidewire is removed and replaced with a 260-cm Super Stiff Amplatz wire (Cook), which is passed into the external carotid artery. The JB2 catheter is removed, and the fluoroscope is panned in the anterior-posterior position from the cervical carotid artery across the arch to allow assessment of the angle and origin of the great vessel. The operator should observe the angle of the vessels carefully; an angle that is too acute at the carotid or innominate artery junction may kink the delivery sheath. Conversion to the open approach may be appropriate when vessel angles are deemed too acute.

When the arch anatomy is favorable, a flexible delivery catheter such as the Flexor catheter by Cook is inserted into the midcarotid position, the Amplatz wire is removed, and a 0.014-in. Roadrunner wire is passed across the lesion in the internal carotid artery. Contrast is injected for road mapping, and the dimensions of the artery and the nature and length of the lesion are determined. In some cases, a stent can be deployed without ballooning. When ballooning is required, a small-sized balloon (4 mm × 2 cm) with a 120-cm shaft length is selected and passed to the lesion. When atropine has been administered, the balloon is inflated for a few seconds at 8–10 atmospheres. At this point in the procedure, a small bolus of contrast is injected to assess the angioplasty result.

Once a stent has been selected and passed to the lesion, a second contrast bolus is injected to confirm proper location. The stent is deployed using a 5-sec balloon inflation in the case of the Palmaz stent. The self-expanding Wallstent is released quickly into the vessel. If there is any

question regarding proper deployment, an intravascular ultrasound study is performed. If deployment is adequate, a
final control angiogram that includes the intracranial circulation is performed. As mentioned previously, it may be
advantageous to image at baseline (before any manipulation) for comparison with the control study. When deployment is not adequate, additional dilation of the stent with
a larger balloon is performed.

After dilation, the guiding catheter is withdrawn into
the descending thoracic aorta and a short 9F sheath is sub-
stituted in the groin. The patient is then transferred to the
intensive care unit for observation and duplex scanning.
The groin sheath is removed when the ACT returns to normal. The primary complication associated with femoral access is groin hematoma; careful sheath removal and attention to the patient's coagulation status are preventive
measures. Pseudoaneurysm and arteriovenous fistula are
also potential complications but are relatively uncommon.

IV. DISCUSSION

At the Arizona Heart Institute, our carotid stenting program
includes only those patients in whom we believe the benefits of the endoluminal intervention potentially outweigh
the risks. While the majority of our experience involves lesions in the internal carotid, we sometimes see lesions in
two locations, one or both of which may be amenable to endovascular therapy. Combined procedures for dual stenoses may include endarterectomy and angioplasty (20,21).

We have encountered high-grade stenosis of the left
common carotid artery at the aortic arch in combination
with an occlusive process of the left carotid bifurcation.
Treatment of the proximal lesion is required before or in
concert with the more cephalad intervention. In general,
the proximal lesions are easily corrected with stents and
are not particularly prone to embolization. Treatment of bi-

furcation lesions depends on their morphological characteristics; classic endarterectomy should be employed in friable lesions with loose debris.

Changes in both patient selection and technique have dramatically reduced the incidence of complications at our center. Analysis of results in a current series of 179 patients indicates a procedural success rate of 96% and a 3.6% rate of neurological complications. The overall rate of death and neurological complications declined from 10.9% in our initial series (6) to 6.2% in the current series.

Of the three deaths in the current series, one was clearly preventable. The patient had an open exposure of the carotid artery for internal carotid artery stenting. Shortly after she was returned to the ICU, her blood pressure increased suddenly to nearly 300 mmHg systolic. Swelling in her neck caused tracheal compression, and she arrested despite a tracheotomy. The second death occurred in a patient who received an Integra stent (investigational device; Boston Scientific/Meadox) and died from distal embolization. A third patient died several hours after the procedure from a distal dissection of the internal carotid artery that occurred well above the location of the stent and resulted in complete thrombosis of the artery.

Indeed, there are major differences in complication rates and postprocedural results, depending on the exact location of the intervention. The potential for periprocedural embolization is undoubtedly greatest in lesions at the level of the carotid bifurcation. Loose atherosclerotic debris is frequently present here, and passing a wire and balloon and deploying a stent under these circumstances may dislodge it. The results of our current series are impressive given that a subset of patients had combined lesions. Had classic surgical intervention been used, it is doubtful that comparable results could have been obtained.

Restenosis has proven to be a major limitation of angioplasty and stenting in other vessels but, as yet, there are no comprehensive studies of incidence in patients who have undergone carotid procedures. Thus far, our own experience indicates that the restenosis rate in carotid lesions treated with angioplasty and stenting has been quite low. In a large, international, multicenter registry, the restenosis rate was less than 5% at 6 months (10).

V. CONCLUSIONS

Treatment of carotid occlusive disease always involves the risk of embolization and neurological complications. The potential for problems is particularly great in treating occlusive disease at the bifurcation, where lesions may be unusually friable. The development of low-profile devices has improved access and reduced the potential for complications, and noninvasive imaging with intravascular ultrasound and duplex imaging have made carotid procedures safer and more effective.

Although our experience with endovascular intervention at the carotid bifurcation is limited, early results indicate reasonable technical success. Rates of neurological complications with endovascular procedures do appear to be somewhat higher than those associated with endarterectomy; angioplasty and stenting may be most appropriate in patients who are predisposed to surgical complications. Cost containment of endovascular intervention will be an important part of introducing the technology into wider use.

REFERENCES

1. Kachel R, Basche S, Heerklotz I, Grossmann K, Endler S. Percutaneous transluminal angioplasty of supra-aortic arteries, especially the internal carotid artery. Neuroradiology 1991; 33:191–194.
2. Kachel R. Results of balloon angioplasty in the carotid arteries. J Endovasc Surg 1996; 3:22–30.

3. Theron J. Angioplastie carotidienne protegee et stents carotidiens. J Mal Vasc 1996; 21(suppl A):113–22.

4. Gaines P. The European carotid angioplasty trial (abstr). J Endovasc Surg 1996; 3:107.

5. Gaines PA. Carotid angioplasty and CAVATAS update (abstr). J Endovasc Surg 1997; 4(suppl 1):I12.

6. Diethrich EB, Ndiaye M, Reid DB. Stenting in the carotid artery: initial experience in 110 patients. J Endovasc Surg 1996; 3:42–62.

7. Iyer SS, Roubin G, Yadav S, Vitek J, Parks JM, Wadlington V, Doblar D, Jordan W. Elective carotid stenting (abstr). J Endovasc Surg 1996; 3:105–106.

8. Wholey MH, Wholey M, Jarmolowski CR, Eles G, Levy D, Buecthel J. Endovascular stents for carotid artery occlusive disease. J Endovasc Surg 1997; 4:326–338.

9. Teitlebaum GP, Lefkowitz MA, Giannotta SL. Carotid angioplasty and stenting in high-risk patients. Surg Neurol 1998; 50:300–311.

10. Wholey MH, Wholey M, Bergeron P, Diethrich EB, Henry M, Laborde JC, Mathias K, Myla S, Roubin GS, Shawl F, Theron JG, Yadav JS, Dorros G, Guimaraens J, Higashida R, Kumar V, Leon M, Lim M, Londero H, Mesa J, Ramee S, Rodriguez A, Rosenfield K, Teitlebaum G, Vozzi C. Current global status of carotid artery stent placement. Cathet Cardicvasc Diagn 1998; 44:1–6.

11. Jordan WD Jr, Voellinger DC, Doblar DD Plyushcheva NP, Fisher WS, McDowell HA. Microemboli detected by transcranial Doppler monitoring in patients during carotid angioplasty versus carotid endarterectomy. Cardiovasc Surg 1999; 7:33–38.

12. Jordan WD Jr, Schroeder PT, Fisher WS, McDowell HA. A comparison of angioplasty with stenting versus endarterectomy for the treatment of carotid artery stenosis. Ann Vasc Surg 1997; 11:2–8.

13. Jordan WD Jr, Roye GD, Fisher WS 3rd, Redden D, McDowell HA. A cost comparison of balloon angioplasty and stenting versus endarterectomy for the treatment of carotid artery stenosis. J Vasc Surg 1998; 27:16–22.

14. National Stroke Association. Current status of carotid stenting. Stroke Clin Update 1999; 9:1–4.

15. Hobson RW 2nd, Brott T, Ferguson R, Roubin G, Moore W, Kuntz R, Howard G, Ferguson J. CREST: carotid revascularization endarterectomy versus stent trial. Cardiovasc Surg 1997; 5:457–458.
16. Wholey MH. Randomizing carotid endarterectomy to carotid stenting? J Endovasc Surg 1999; 6:127–129.
17. Kharrazi MR. Anesthesia for carotid stent procedures. J Endovasc Surg 1996; 3:211–216.
18. Bergeron P, Chamabran P, Benichou H, et al, Recurrent carotid disease: will stents be an alternative to surgery? J Endovasc Surg 1996; 3:76–79.
19. Alessandri C, Bergeron P. Local anesthesia in carotid angioplasty. J Endovasc Surg 1996; 3:31–34.
20. Levien LJ, Benn CA, Veller MG, Fritz VU. Retrograde balloon angioplasty of brachiocephalic or common carotid artery stenoses at the time of carotid endarterectomy. Eur J Vasc Endovasc Surg 1998; 15:521–527.
21. Sidhu PS, Morgan MB, Walters HL, Baskerville PA, Fraser SC. Technical report: Combined carotid bifrucation endarterectomy and intraoperative transluminal angioplasty of a proximal common carotid artery stenosis: an alternative to extrathoracic bypass. Clin Radiol 1998; 53:444–447.

8

Endovascular Management of Carotid Artery Stenosis

The Impact of Cerebral Protection

Michel Henry, Max Amor, Christos Klonaris, Isabelle Henry, and Michèle Hugel
U.C.C.I. Polyclinique d'Essey, Essey-les-Nancy, France

Cerebrovascular disease remains a major public health problem. It is the third leading cause of death and accounts for approximately 150,000 strokes per year in France and 500,000 strokes per year in the United States (1,2). Carotid artery stenosis accounts for 20–30% of all cases (2). The incidence of the ischemic origin of stroke increases with age, being 80% after age 50 (3). A program of preventive therapy and treatment of carotid artery stenosis is therefore necessary.

Recent results of multicenter randomized trials proved the superiority of carotid endarterectomy (CEA) over medical treatment for both asymptomatic and symptomatic patients and better clarified the indications for surgery (4–8). However, the inherent risks of surgery limit the application of CEA. The risk of periprocedural stroke was 5.8% in the NASCET study, 7.5% in the ECST study, and 2.3% in the ACAS study. Despite the fact that endarterectomies were performed by experienced surgeons in these studies, high-risk patients were excluded. Patients with associated significant coronary artery disease represent a particularly high-risk group for postoperative neurological and cardiac events (4,9). Other complications of CEA include cranial nerve palsies (7.6–27%) (4–11), neck hematomas (5.5%) (4), and restenosis (5–9%) (12,13). Rothwell et al. (14) studied 50 surgical series and found the risk of cerebrovascular accidents to be 2.3% in the series with surgical follow-up, but 7.7% in the series followed by neurologists.

Based on the results from various national and international trials, the Ad Hoc Committee of the AHA proposed specific guidelines to perform carotid endarterectomy (15). Indications were divided into proven, acceptable but not proven, uncertain, and proven inappropriate and further stratified according to patients' status. Asymptomatic and symptomatic patients should have a combined morbidity and mortality rate less than 3% and 6%, respectively, to maintain the beneficial effects of endarterectomy over medical treatment. To consider carotid angioplasty as an alternative to surgery, its complication rate should parallel that of endarterectomy.

Percutaneous techniques have proved their efficacy in the coronary and peripheral circulations and therefore may also be proposed for extracranial carotid artery stenosis. Several recent studies evaluated the role of angioplasty and stenting in the carotid territory. Experienced operators can now obtain combined stroke and death rates less than 5%, similar to surgical results (16–22). However, endovascular treatment is still not widely accepted for carotid artery stenosis. Interventionists have been reluctant mainly due to the potential risks of cerebral embolism during the steps of the procedure. Indeed the majority of the reported neurological complications are due to the intracerebral embolism of plaque fragments or thrombus. The concept of cerebral protection during angioplasty and the applicability of suitable devices may open new avenues in the endovascular treatment of carotid artery stenosis, minimizing the embolic risk and complication rate, widening the indications for the procedure. In this review we are reporting our personal experience with carotid artery angioplasty and stenting both with and without cerebral protection in a series of more than 300 patients.

I. AUTHORS' EXPERIENCE

A. Population

From April 1995 to August 1999, 334 carotid angioplasty procedures were attempted (right: 157, left: 177) in 308 patients (males: 225, mean age 70.5 ± 9.6 years). Fifty-six percent of the patients were asymptomatic. Twenty-six patients underwent bilateral procedures. Major risk factors were hypertension in 63%, diabetes in 26%, dyslipidemia in 50%, and smoking in 61%. Associated diseases were coronary artery disease in 55%, peripheral vascular disease in 34%, pulmonary insufficiency in 8%, and renal insufficiency in 5% of the patients. Sixty-five percent of them would have been excluded definitely or temporarily from the NASCET or ACAS studies. All were required to sign an informed consent statement.

B. Lesion Assessment

We routinely performed two studies before the procedure.

Echodoppler

This examination allowed us to assess the localization, morphology, and degree of the stenosis, and the presence of calcification or plaque ulceration. A characterization of plaque echogenicity was also made. A transcranial Doppler study completed the examination.

Angiography

We used intra-arterial DSA with at least two orthogonal projections of the carotid bifurcation. Intracranial images were routinely obtained to detect the status of collateral circulation and the presence of intracranial stenosis or vascular malformation that may contraindicate angioplasty or require another interventional procedure. Most of the lesions were atheromatous ($n = 300$), 26 were restenoses, 17 developed after endarterectomy, and nine developed following angioplasty. Seven lesions were related to radiation injury, and one was a posttraumatic aneurysm. The mean diameter of the internal carotid artery was 5.3 ± 1.2 mm as determined by the quantitative carotid analysis method. To calculate the degree of stenosis we used the NASCET angiographic criteria (4) before and after angioplasty and stenting. Mean stenosis was $82.3 \pm 8.7\%$. Ulceration was found in 178 lesions (53.2%). Contralateral carotid stenosis was present in 55 and occlusion in 16 cases. The bifurcation was involved in 130 cases, isolated common carotid artery stenosis were observed in 11 cases, and three patients had separate lesions in both common and internal carotid arteries.

C. Neurological Assessment

Neurological assessment was performed by an independent neurologist before and at 24 hrs, 30 days, and 6 months after the procedure using the N-Score examination scale for middle cerebral artery infarction (23). Baseline CT scan or MRI was also obtained, and abnormalities were detected in 28% of the asymptomatic patients.

D. The Procedure

Technique

Angioplasty without cerebral protection (Figs. 1, 2) was performed in 166 cases mainly at the beginning of our practice. The femoral access was most often used (151 cases). The common carotid artery was first catheterized with a Side-winder catheter (Cordis, a Johnson & Johnson Co., Warren, NJ). An 8F or 9F guiding catheter was then placed in the common carotid artery directly or mounted on a rigid Amplatz 0.035-in. guidewire previously placed in the external carotid to maintain good support. Baseline images of the lesion and intracranial circulation were performed. We then usually used a 3-mm-long 0.018-in. coronary guidewire (Roadrunner, Cook France, Charenton Cedex) to cross the lesion cautiously to eliminate embolic events. The stenosis was usually predilated with a small diameter (3.5 or 4 mm) coronary dilatation catheter. We generally used a Speedy Bypass balloon (Schneider, Bülach, Switzerland). The inflation was of short duration to facilitate stent passage. Next, a stent was placed to cover the lesion and dilated in a diameter equal to that of the artery. In a few cases, it was not possible to selectively catheterize the carotid artery using the femoral approach due to severe arterial tortuosity. When this approach was contraindicated, we utilized

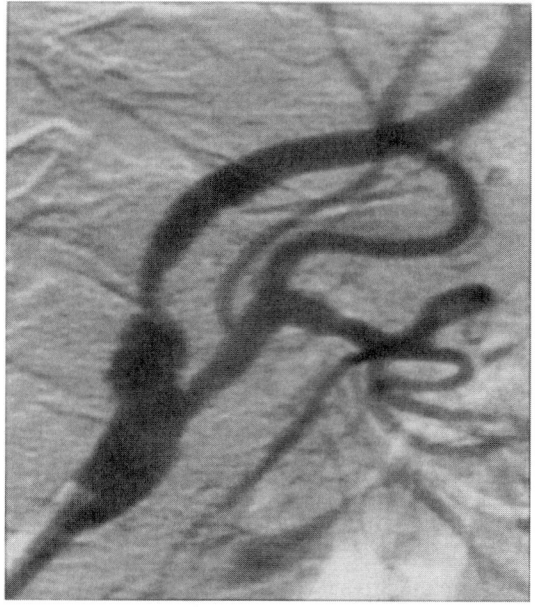

(a)

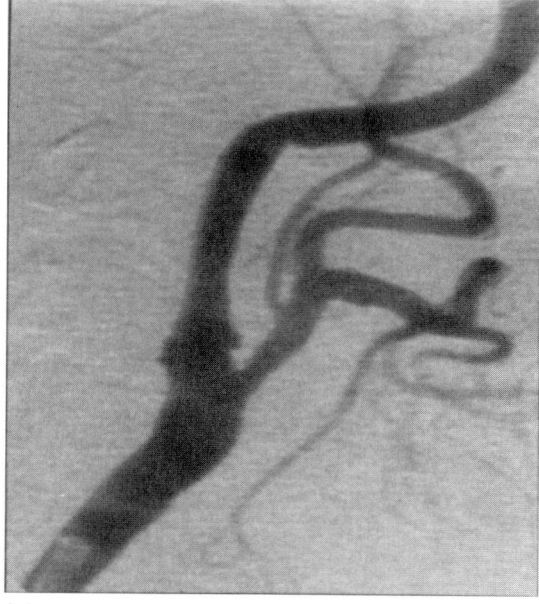

(b)

direct carotid artery puncture (13 cases) and the brachial approach (2 cases).

Angioplasty with cerebral protection was performed in 168 arteries.

Theron's Technique (24). We used this technique in 47 patients at the beginning of our experience with protection devices. It consisted of using a triple coaxial catheter that occluded the internal carotid artery beyond the stenosis with a latex balloon. Angioplasty and stent placement were then performed under cerebral protection. Any generated debris was aspirated through the guiding catheter placed in the internal carotid artery. A flush toward the external carotid artery followed the aspiration. We observed four complications with this technique and subsequently we no longer used it. We found some disadvantages: the device has poor radiopacity and the catheter is not steerable; in at least 10% of the cases it is not possible to cross the lesion, and there is a risk of dislodging a plaque when crossing the stenosis (one case in our series).

The PercuSurge Guardwire Temporary Occlusion and Aspiration System. This is the technique we now routinely use. The device (PercuSurge Inc., Sunnyvale, CA) consists of several components. The Guardwire is a 0.014-in. or 0.018-in. angioplasty wire (190 and 300 cm in length) constructed of hollow nitinol hypotube. Incorporated into the distal wire segment is an inflatable elastomeric balloon capable of occluding vessel outflow. The proximal end of the hypotube wire incorporates a Microseal allowing inflation and deflation of the occlusion balloon utilizing a Microseal adapter. The Guardwire is advanced through the guiding catheter previously placed into the common carotid artery, and after crossing the lesion the occlusion balloon is placed distal to

---

Figure 1 (a) Severe right internal carotid artery symptomatic stenosis. (b) Satisfactory result after angioplasty and stent placement.

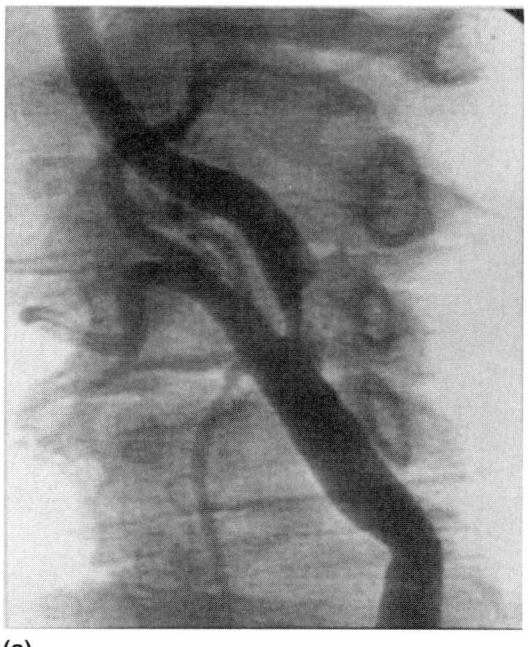

(a)

Figure 2   (a) Severe ulcerated stenosis of a left internal carotid artery. (b) Lesion predilation and stenting under protection with the PercuSurge device. The distal (cephalad) marker corresponds to the inflated occlusion balloon, the proximal marker to the tip of the aspiration catheter. (c) Final result.

the stenosis. The Microseal adapter is attached and the balloon is slowly inflated with a fixed volume of dilute contrast occluding internal carotid artery outflow. Upon detaching the Microseal adapter, the balloon remains inflated; thus angioplasty and stenting are performed under protection. An aspiration catheter is then advanced over the wire into the vessel and manual suction is applied to retrieve any generated debris. A flushing can be performed thereafter through this aspiration catheter or the guiding catheter directing the flow toward the external carotid artery. The Mi-

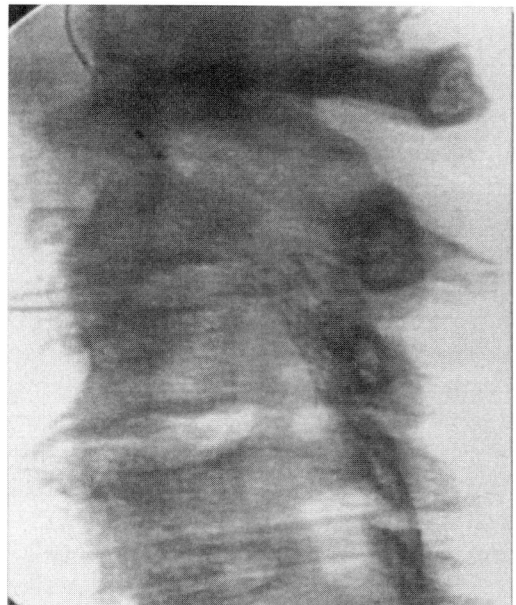

(b)

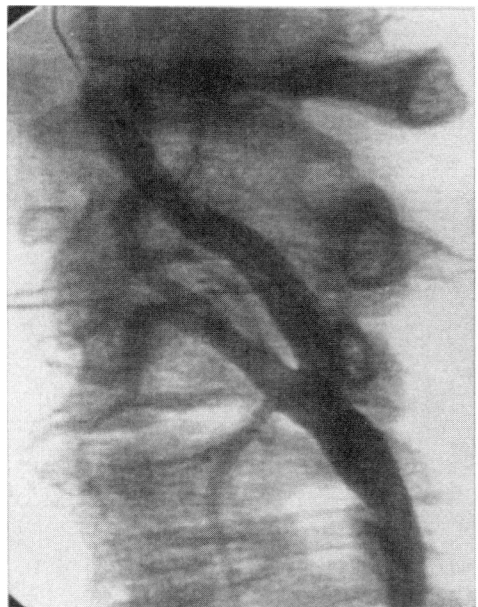

(c)

croseal adapter is then reattached to the Guardwire and the distal occlusion balloon is deflated, allowing normal vessel flow to resume. Two techniques can be used: the occlusion balloon could remain inflated during the total procedure or it could be deflated between predilation and stenting. In the second case, two aspirations ± flushing should be done, after predication and after stenting. We have initiated the first clinical study and attempted to treat 111 lesions in 100 patients. We observed technical success in 110 arteries (99.1%). In one case it was impossible to cross the lesion with the Guardwire due to severe tortuosity of the common and internal carotid artery.

Tolerance to occlusion balloon was satisfactory in 104 cases (95%). One patient with poor collateral circulation developed complete intolerance with loss of consciousness and seizures rapidly after balloon inflation. In that case we had to deflate the balloon and the procedure was continued without cerebral protection. The patient had uneventful recovery immediately after balloon deflation. Five patients had transient intolerance manifested by agitation and impaired verbal communication, starting approximately 2 min after the protection balloon was inflated. This resolved quickly before the end of the procedure. A hypotensive episode during lesion dilatation was a probable precipitating factor in two patients. Additionally three patients developed vasospasm distal to the stenosis, but this recovered rapidly with vasodilator therapy.

The mean balloon occlusion time was 470 ± 220 sec (125–1479 sec). Visible debris was removed with the aspiration catheter in all patients and analyzed. The number of particles varied from seven to 283 per procedure, mean 78 particles per procedure. The mean diameter of recovered particles was 270 μ (56–2846 μ). Debris was composed of atheromatous plaques, necrotic core, cholesterol crystals, fibrin, organized or fresh thrombi, lipid masses, platelets, and macrophage foam cells. With this technique we observed one periprocedural ischemic neurological deficit (0.9%), an amaurosis after an acute thrombosis of a wall stent, which was treated with Reopro. This appeared after flushing toward the external carotid artery in a patient with an anastomosis between the external and internal carotid arteries.

The Medicorp, Henry-Amor-Frid-Rüfenacht (H.A.F.R.) Device. We have developed a new cerebral protection device that consists of: (1) a long hemostatic valve sheath, which is advanced into the common carotid artery, and (2) a microcatheter with a compliant protection balloon fixed at its tip, with markers on its center for good radiological localization. This microcatheter is mounted over a steerable 0.014-in. coronary guidewire, which is first placed in the internal carotid artery and maintained there during the whole procedure, providing a maximum of safety for all potential balloon exchanges. Next a dilatation balloon is advanced over the microcatheter and placed after inflation of the protection balloon. A balloon-expandable stent is placed over the dilatation balloon. If the stent is self-expandable, it is directly advanced over the microcatheter, without lesion predilatation. Angioplasty and stenting are performed under cerebral protection. Debris and particles generated are flushed toward the external carotid artery and/or aspirated. The advantage of this technique is that any coronary-steerable or hydrophilic guidewire may be used according to the type of the lesion. The device is quite radiopaque, thus avoiding certain problems encountered with Theron's technique. We have started the first clinical study and treated 10 patients with success. It seems to have the same advantages as the PercuSurge device.

Stents Used

Stents were deployed in all patients but one. Two stent types were used in the majority of the cases: Palmaz stents

P154–P204, (Cordis/J&J, Warren, NJ) were placed in 199 arteries (211 stents). These stents were chosen mainly for lesions located above the bifurcation. For lesions involving the bifurcation, Wallstent (Boston Scientific, Natick, MA) stents were implanted in 77 arteries, for complete covering. Thirty-four nitinol self-expandable Expander stents (Medicorp, Villers-les-Nancy, France) were implanted in 31 arteries. We also deployed 10 nitinol self-expandable Smart stents (Cordis/J&J, Warren, NJ), one covered Jomed stent (Jomed France SARL, Voisins le Bretonneux) to treat an aneurysm, and 12 other stent types. Seventy-five stents were placed without preliminary dilatation in easily crossable lesions.

Medications, Monitoring, and Follow-up of the Patients

All patients received aspirin 250 mg/day and Ticlopidine 250 to 500 mg/day, or Clopidogrel 75 mg/day for at least two days prior to the procedure. Before the procedure, an intravenous bolus of 5000 IU of unfractionated heparin and 1 mg of atropine were administered. Heparin was continued at therapeutic doses (ACT > 200 sec) until the following day and antiplatelet therapy was given alone thereafter. In five patients with subocclusive ulcerated lesions, abciximab (bolus and continuous infusion) was empirically given during and after the procedure. All patients were cautiously and constantly monitored, and significant changes in pulse rate and blood pressure during dilation and stent placement were corrected immediately.

On day 1, all patients underwent an echodoppler, a CT scan, and a neurological examination. An angiogram was performed only if a particular problem was suspected. At day 30, an echodoppler and neurological examination were performed. At 6 months, an angiogram was systematically performed, along with an echodoppler and neurological examination. The patients were thereafter followed by an echodoppler examination every 6 months. An angiogram was performed only if restenosis was suspected.

Study End-Points

Primary clinical end-points were any postprocedural neurological deficit, myocardial infarction, or death that occurred during or within the first 30 days of the procedure, as well as the need for a new intervention, angioplasty, or endarterectomy at 6 months. Angiographic end-points were technical success rate, defined as achieving a <30% residual stenosis, and restenosis on the follow-up angiogram at 6 months, defined as a reduction of arterial lumen diameterly more than 50%.

E. Results

Immediate Results

Balloon dilatation and stent placement were successful in all patients but one. Due to severe arterial tortuosity in one case, it was impossible to selectively catheterize the right common carotid artery. The mean residual stenosis after the procedure was 2.9 ± 7%. Ultrasound examination at 24 h and angiography when performed showed excellent arterial patency in all patients.

Complications

We observed 13 periprocedural ischemic neurological complications (3.9%): four transient ischemic attacks (1.2%), two of them in patients older than 79 years; four minor strokes (1.2%) with transient hemiparesis—the consecutive CT scans (days 1, 3, 7) never revealed any particular lesion; five major strokes (1.5%): two amaurosis, one with Theron's technique, one with the PercuSurge device, and three hemiplegias, one despite Theron's technique. One patient with hemiplegia died a week later; another patient died at 3 weeks from cardiac failure. Additionally one minor stroke due to an intracerebral hemorrhage appeared on the third postoperative day after treatment of a tight internal carotid artery stenosis under cerebral protection with PercuSurge and Reopro. This resolved within 5 days.

Eight complications appeared after Palmaz stent implantation (4%) and four after Wallstent (5.2%). Five appeared in the presence of asymptomatic lesions (2.8%) and eight in symptomatic lesions (5.8%). Five complications, including three major strokes, appeared during the first 60 procedures ($p < 0.05$). Eight (4.8%) appeared during carotid angioplasty and stenting performed without cerebral protection, five despite cerebral protection (3%) ($p < 0.05$). Among these were four with Theron's technique (8.5%) and one with the PercuSurge technique (0.9%) ($p < 0.01$) (Table 1). Excellent patency of the carotid artery was seen in all cases. Local complications consisted of three cervical hematomas that appeared after direct puncture of the carotid artery and required surgery.

Follow-up

At 6 months nine patients died from procedure-unrelated causes; 220 had a follow-up by either angiography (155) or a duplex scan (65) examination. We reported one mild com-

Table 1 Neurological Complications After Carotid Angioplasty

	Unprotected ($n = 166$)	Protected ($n = 168$)
Major stroke	2	3
Minor stroke	3	1
TIA	3	1
Total	8 (4.8%)	5 (3%) $p < 0.05$
Theron's technique		4/47 (8.5%)
PercuSurge technique		1/111 (0.9%) $p < 0.01$
H.A.F.R. technique		0/10

pression of a Palmaz stent without significant stenosis and 11 restenoses (5%). One patient had a transient ischemic accident; he was successfully treated by a second angioplasty. The remaining 10 restenoses were asymptomatic. One severe silent restenosis with a reduction of the lumen by 85% occurred after migration of a Wallstent stent into the common carotid artery. A new angioplasty and stenting was performed with excellent result. Seven restenoses were also treated by another angioplasty. One silent thrombosis of the internal carotid artery within the stent was treated medically. One restenosis occurred in a Viktor stent and could not be redilated. This patient was treated by surgery with a good result. Also, one external carotid artery was thrombosed after Palmaz stent implantation. This vessel remained patent in all other cases.

The mean follow-up was 17.1 ± 8.5 months (maximum 53 months). A total of 185 patients were followed without any new neurological event or restenosis. Twelve procedure-unrelated deaths occurred. The primary patency at 4 years was 96% and the secondary patency was 99%.

II. DISCUSSION

Our results have shown that carotid angioplasty with stent placement may be performed with a complication rate that is not higher than that of surgery despite the fact that a large number of high-risk patients were included. The major neurological complication rate was 1.5%, and the minor neurological complication rate was 2.4%.

Several authors reported favorable results using interventional techniques. Diethrich et al. (16) in their series of 110 patients reported seven cerebrovascular accidents (6.4%) (two major, five minor) and five transient ischemic attacks (4.5%). Roubin et al. (17) reported one death, two major strokes, and seven minor strokes, five of them with complete recovery, in treating 152 carotid stenoses with

stenting. Recently, Mathias (18) presented his data. Since
1989, 799 internal carotid artery stenoses exceeding 70%
were treated in 633 patients. Angioplasty alone was used
in 32.7% and stenting in 67.3% of the procedures. The
death rate was 0.4% (two patients) and neurological complications included transient ischemic accidents in 4.4%, minor stroke in 1.6%, and a major stroke in 0.9%. Wholey et
al. (19) reported data from 114 procedures with successful
Palmaz stent implantation in 108 arteries. Complications
included two major strokes, two minor strokes, and five
transient ischemic accidents. Strokes seem to happen more
often in patients with bradycardia and hypotension generated by the pressure exerted on the carotid bulb baroreceptors by balloon dilatation (25). Bradycardia and hypotension reduce cerebral blood flow, leading to ischemia in
patients dependent on collateral flow. Prompt use of atropine and right heart pacing are important to avoid the risk
of cerebral hypoperfusion.

III. RATIONALE FOR BRAIN PROTECTION

All the above data show that in the hands of experienced
interventionists, the morbidity and mortality rates of carotid angioplasty and stenting combined are low, comparable to surgical results. However, the risk of embolic events
remains during the procedure; different steps may dislodge
embolic particles. This is unpredictable and could occur at
any time: with placement of the guiding catheter in the
common carotid artery, when crossing the lesion with
guidewires, balloons, or stents, during balloon dilatation of
the lesion, and during stent implantation and dilatation,
which is considered the most embolic step of the procedure.
In a large carotid endarterectomy study, Riles et al. (25)
found that postoperative thromboses and emboli were responsible for 40% of the strokes. In a similar fashion, mi-
croembolization and thrombosis due to platelet aggregation

account for the majority of strokes after carotid angioplasty and stenting (19). Several authors (24,26–28) using different methods have found evidence of embolic particles. The clinical significance of the number of embolic particles generated is not clear. Intuition leads one to believe that patients in whom balloon angioplasty and stenting produce a higher number and larger particles would be expected to have a higher periprocedural stroke rate than patients in whom fewer or smaller particles are produced (28). These particles consist of atherosclerotic debris, organized thrombi, and calcified material. There is a correlation with the number of particles and carotid stenoses greater than 90% and with echolucent plaques (28), advanced age, lesion severity, and long and multiple lesions (29).

Stent implantation probably contributes to the reduction of procedural complications and currently it seems that routine stenting is accepted by the majority of investigators, independent of angioplasty results. But stenting itself is not a sufficient method to protect from cerebral embolism. The choice of the stent is still an open issue. Two of the most frequently implanted stents, the Palmaz stent and the Wallstent, have specific advantages and limitations (17,19,30,31). Unfortunately, the perfect stent does not yet exist and improvements in stent technology are necessary. It is expected that the new generation of nitinol stents, specifically designed for the carotid artery, will improve the results of the technique.

Neurological complication rates could be reduced by the use of a cerebral protection devices. Vitec et al., in 1984, reported a case of successful innominate artery angioplasty where the risk of cerebral embolization was reduced by temporary occlusion of the origin of the right common carotid artery with a second balloon catheter (32). In the last decade several protective techniques have been proposed during carotid angioplasty.

(1) The technique described by Kachel (21) is based on occlusion of the common carotid artery after dilatation of

the lesion but before balloon deflation, followed by aspiration, thus limiting the risks of cerebral embolization. In his series, Kachel reported a neurological complication rate of 4.6%, which does not seem lower than the complication rates of several series without cerebral protection. (2) With the technique described by Theron et al. (24) in their series of 136 cases, no embolization was reported during angioplasty with cerebral protection, but two embolic complications occurred, one during placement of a Strecker stent and the other 6 h after the procedure. (3) The two new techniques of cerebral protection used, derived from Theron's technique, seem safer and easier to use. Their most important advantage is the possibility of crossing the lesion with a coronary guidewire. We have treated 111 lesions with the PercuSurge device and 10 with our device and we observed only one neurological complication related to this technique itself. We did not randomize our patients to undergo standard or protected angioplasty; in addition, unprotected angioplasties were performed almost entirely in our early experience. However, concerning embolic events, our results reached statistical and clinical significance in favor of protected techniques, despite disappointing results with Theron's technique. (4) Filter devices—guidewire-based devices with a nitinol basket attached at the distal end—are currently in development or early clinical use. It is too early to assess whether they will provide advantages over balloon protection systems. We predict that distal protection devices may play an important role in future carotid angioplasty and stenting procedures.

IV. INDICATIONS

The indications for endovascular treatment of carotid artery stenosis are still much debated and no consensus has yet appeared. Several indications seem to be well accepted now: 1) patients presenting high surgical risk (elderly patients, patients with severe cardiopulmonary disorders that preclude general anesthesia or a prolonged surgical procedure, and patients with severe renal insufficiency), 2) patients with a surgical restenosis, particularly early, when it is usually associated with intimal hyperplasia, 3) postradiation carotid stenosis, 4) high bifurcation at or near the base of the skull that would require dislocation of the mandible for surgical exposure, 5) distal lesions located in the distal internal carotid artery, including fibromuscular dysplasia, 6) proximal or carotid-ostial lesions. However, particularly when performed under cerebral protection, the indications of carotid angioplasty could be broader depending on the symptomatic or asymptomatic status of the patients. In the presence of symptoms, all patients with a stenosis ≥70% could be candidates for carotid angioplasty and stenting. In the presence of an asymptomatic stenosis, the indications are more difficult. We know that the benefits of surgery are very low, and currently it has not yet been proven that stenting is comparable to surgery in terms of long-term results. The criteria for intervention derived from the ACAS study seem too broad to us. We prefer to limit our indications as follows: 1) stenosis more than 75/80%, 2) rapidly progressive stenosis on two consecutive echodoppler examinations, 3) bilateral tight stenoses, 4) stenoses presenting specific characteristics on the echodoppler. The incidence of CT brain infarcts and transcranial Doppler embolic counts are increased with increasing plaque echolucency (25).

Three patients with pedunculated thrombi of the internal carotid artery were refused angioplasty and were referred for surgery. These lesions are not considered suitable for angioplasty since the risk of embolism seems to be very high; surgery is therefore the preferred treatment.

There are several advantages of carotid angioplasty over surgery. It is performed through a percutaneous access under local anesthesia, which allows for strict monitoring of the patient throughout the entire procedure. It can be proposed in high-risk patients and allows treatment of lesions that cannot be accessed with surgery. A combined carotid-coronary percutaneous revascularization can be performed. Sixteen percent of the patients in Yadav's series (20) benefited from such procedures. One should keep in mind that surgical interventions combining carotid endarterectomy and coronary bypass lead to cerebrovascular accidents ranging from 4.5 to 7.1% and to a mortality rate of 5.4–5.7% (25). Carotid bifurcation stenting allows for treatment of lesions of the supra-aortic vessels during the same procedure. The duration of cerebral ischemia due to dilatation or inflation of the protection balloon is short. Surgical clamping can last from 20 to 40 min, and placement of a shunt can last from 2 to 3 min. Surgical restenoses, with operative risk, in some series, much higher than that of de novo endarterectomy, can be treated more easily by angioplasty. The absence of a surgical incision avoids numerous local complications such as nerve injuries, infections, and hematomas, as seen in 2–12.5% of post-carotid endarterectomy cases. Hospital stays may be shorter, with discharge at 24–48 hr after the procedure.

V. CONCLUSION

Carotid angioplasty and stent implantation currently seems to be a reliable and efficient method. The risks do not seem greater than those of surgery, and the procedure addresses high-risk patients with contraindications to a surgical intervention. However, this technique is difficult and it should be performed by well-trained, multidisciplinary teams. Certain indications are already well accepted and will probably enlarge thanks to improvements in techniques, notably better stents and new methods of cerebral protection.

We believe that cerebral protection will probably extend to all cerebral angioplasty procedures. It will likely widen the indications and produce complication rates lower than those obtained with surgery, particularly for lesions with high embolic risks. One may also wonder whether it is sensible to initiate larger randomized studies, particularly versus surgery, without cerebral protection techniques since their utilization may lead to improved results. Beginners should wait for these techniques to make their procedures maximally safe.

REFERENCES

1. Mellière D. Chirurgie carotidienne: bilan et problèmes actuels. J Mal Vasc 1993; 18:176–185.
2. De Bakey ME Carotid endarterectomy revisited. J Endovasc Surg 1996; 3:4.
3. Boosser MG, Mas JC. Epidémiologie des accidents vasculaires cérébraux du sujet jeune. Presse Med 1988; 17:143–145.
4. North American Symptomatic Carotid Endarterectomy Trial Collaborators. Beneficial effect of carotid endarterectomy in symptomatic patients with high-grade carotid stenosis. N Engl J Med 1991; 325:445–453.
5. North American Symptomatic Carotid Endarterectomy Trial Collaborators. Benefit of carotid endarterectomy in patients with symptomatic moderate or severe stenosis. N Engl J Med 1998; 339:1415–1425.
6. European Carotid Surgery Trialists' Collaborative Group. MRC European Carotid Surgery Trial: interim results for symptomatic patients with severe (70–99%) or with mild (0–29%) carotid stenosis. Lancet 1991; 337:1235–1243.
7. European Carotid Surgery Trialists Collaborative Group. Randomized trial of endarterectomy for recently symptomatic carotid stenosis: final results of the MRC European Carotid Study Trial (ECST). Lancet 1998; 351:1379–1387.
8. The Executive Committee for the Asymptomatic Carotid Atherosclerosis Study. Endarterectomy for asymptomatic carotid artery stenosis. JAMA 1995; 273:1421–1428.
9. Winslow CM, Solomon DH, Chassin MR, Kosecoff J, Merrick NJ, Brook RH. The appropriateness of carotid endarterectomy. N Engl J Med. 1988; 318:721–727.

10. Lusby RJ, Wylie EJ. Complications of carotid endarterectomy. Surg Clin North Am 1983; 63:1293–1302.
11. Goldstein LB, Moore WS, Robertson JT, Chaturvedi S. Complication rates for carotid endarterectomy. A call to action. Stroke 1997; 28:889–890.
12. Zierler RE, Brandyk DF, Thiele BL, Strandness DE Jr. Carotid artery stenosis following endarterectomy. Arch Surg 1982; 117:1408–1415.
13. Edwards WH Jr, Edward WH Sr, Mulherin JL Jr, Martin RS III. Recurrent carotid artery stenosis. Resection with autogenous vein replacement Ann Surg 1989; 209:662–669.
14. Rothwell PM, Slattery J, Warlow CP. Systematic comparison of the risks of stroke and death due to carotid endarterectomy for symptomatic and asymptomatic stenosis. Stroke 1996; 27:266–269.
15. Guidelines for carotid endarterectomy: a multidisciplinary consensus statement from the Ad Hoc Committee, American Heart Association. Stroke 1995; 26:188–201.
16. Diethrich EB, Ndiaye M, Reid DB. Stenting in the carotid artery: initial experience in 110 patients. J Endovasc Surg 1996; 3:42–62.
17. Roubin GS, Yadav S, Iyer SS, Vitek J. Carotid stent-supported angioplasty: a neurovascular intervention to prevent stroke. Am J Cardiol 1996; 78(3A):8–12.
18. Mathias KD. Initial and long term results of carotid PTA and stenting: why stent? 11th Annual International Symposium on Endovascular Therapy, Miami, FL, Jan 23–27, 1999.
19. Wholey MH, Wholey M, Jarmolowski CR, Eles G, Levy D, Buecthel J. Endovascular stents for carotid occlusive disease. J Endovasc Surg 1997; 4:326–338.
20. Yadav JS, Roubin GS, Iyers S, Vitek J, King P, Jordan WD, Fisher WS. Elective stenting of the extracranial carotid arteries. Circulation 1997; 95:376–381.
21. Kachel R. Results of balloon angioplasty in the carotid arteries. J Endovasc Surg 1996; 3:22–30.
22. Bergeron P, Chambran P, Bianca S, Benichou H, Massonat J. Traitement endovasculaire des artères à destinée cérébrale: échecs et limites. J Mal Vasc 1996; 21:123–131.
23. Orgogozo JM, Calpideo R, Anagnostou CN, Juge O, Pere JJ, Dartiques JF, Steiner TJ, Yotis A, Rose FC. Mise au point

d'un score neurologique pour l'évaluation clinique des infarctus sylviens. Presse Med 1983; 12:3039–3044.

24. Theron J, Payelle G, Coskun O, Huet HF, Guimaraens L. Carotid artery stenosis: treatment with protected balloon angioplasty and stent placement. Radiology 1996; 201:627–636.
25. Riles TS, Imparato AM, Jacobwitz GR, Lamparello PJ, Gianola G, Adelman MA, Landis R. The cause of perioperative stroke after carotid endarterectomy. J Vasc Surg 1994; 19:206–216.
26. Martin JB, Gailloud P, Sugiu K, Khan H, Spadola L, Piotin M, Fasel JHD, Rufenacht DA. In-vitro models of human carotid atheromatous disease. In Henry M, Amor M, eds. Ninth International Course Book of Peripheral Vascular Intervention, Europa Edition. 1998:541–546.
27. Jordan WD, Voellinger DC, Doblar DD, Plyushcheva NP, Fisher WS, McDowell HA. Microemboli detected by transcranial Doppler monitoring in patients during carotid angioplasty versus carotid endarterectomy. Cardiovasc Surg 1999; 7:33–38.
28. Ohki T, Marin ML, Lyon RT, Berdejo GL, Soundararajan K, Ohki M, Yuan JG, Faries PL, Wain A, Sanchez LA, Suggs WD, Veith FJ. Ex vivo human carotid artery bifurcation stenting: correlation of lesion characteristics with embolic potential. J Vasc Surg 1998; 27:463–471.
29. Mathur A, Roubin GS, Iyer SS, Piamsonboon C, Liu MW, Gomez CR, Yadav JS, Chastain HD, Fox LM, Dean LS, Vitek JJ. Predictors of stroke complicating carotid artery stenting. Circulation 1998; 97:1239–1245.
30. Mathur A, Dorros G, Iyer SS, Vitek JJ, Yadav SS, Roubin GS. Palmaz stent compression in patients following carotid artery stenting. Cathet Cardiovasc Diagn 1997; 41:137–140.
31. Johnson SP, Fujitani RM, Leyendecker JR, Joseph FB. Stent deformation and intimal hyperplasia complicating treatment of a post carotid endarterectomy intimal flap with a Palmaz stent. J Vasc Surg 1997; 25:764–768.
32. Vitek JJ, Raymon BC, Oh SJ. Innominate artery angioplasty. Am J Neuroradiol 1984; 5:113–114.

9

Current Status and Plans for an NIH-Sponsored Clinical Trial of Carotid Bifurcation Angioplasty and Stenting

Robert W. Hobson II
University of Medicine and Dentistry of New Jersey–New Jersey Medical School (NJMS), Newark, New Jersey

I. INTRODUCTION

Carotid bifurcation angioplasty and stenting (CBAS) has been recommended by some clinicians as an alternative to carotid endarterectomy for patients who have extracranial carotid occlusive disease (1–3). However, it should be remembered that carotid endarterectomy is the gold standard and has become the preferred method for treatment of symptomatic and asymptomatic patients with high-grade carotid stenosis, displacing optimal medical management alone as an ethical alternative in managing these patients (1–5). Emergence of a position of clinical equipoise (6) on the relatively equivalent value of these alternatives, as defined by different specialists who manage patients with cerebrovascular insufficiency by different procedures, has resulted in the initiation of a major European clinical trial, Carotid and Vertebral Artery Transluminal Angioplasty Study (CAVATAS) (7), as well as planning in this country for a major effort sponsored by the National Institutes of Health (NIH) (8). Funding has been approved by the National Institute of Neurological Disorders and Stroke (NINDS), and initiation of a randomized clinical trial involving symptomatic extracranial carotid occlusive disease, Carotid Revascularization Endarterectomy Versus Stent Trial (CREST), is planned to begin later this year or early next year. Results of the present consensus conference have confirmed the value of our commitment to a randomized clinical trial to complete an efficacy assessment of CEA versus CBAS.

II. DATA FROM CLINICAL TRIALS

Three (7,9,10) randomized clinical trials comparing the efficacy of CBAS and CEA have been conducted. In Europe, the CAVATAS investigators (17) are comparing surgical intervention and angioplasty for treatment of carotid and vertebral occlusive lesions. Martin Brown, the Principal Investigator of CAVATAS, presented the results from Phase I of his multicenter trial during the American Heart Association's International Stroke meeting in Nashville, Tennessee, in February 1999. Among 504 patients randomized primarily to angioplasty alone or CEA, 30-day disabling stroke and death rates were comparable, 6.3% for CEA and 6.4% for the angioplasty group. Phase II will be initiated later this year and will utilize angioplasty and stenting in all symptomatic carotid cases. These are the only data available on cases randomized to CEA or carotid angioplasty; however, their influence may be blunted by the somewhat higher-than-expected complication rate in the CEA group. A smaller clinical trial (9) was halted prematurely because of a higher-than-expected complication rate in the CBAS arm of the study. However, concerns have been raised as to the investigators' choice of an unacceptably small sample size, inadequate credentialing of the interventionalists performing CBAS, and unrealistic complications from CBAS before the trial was halted and discontinued. Alberts and co-authors (10) described the methodology of another aborted attempt at a randomized clinical trial comparing CBAS and CEA in symptomatic patients (stenoses 50–99%) sponsored by the Schneider Corporation (now Boston Scientific Vascular, manufacturers of the Wallstent endoprosthesis). The stated aim of the trial was to determine whether or not carotid stenting is equivalent to CEA in the prevention of any ipsilateral stroke, periprocedural death (within 30 days), or vascular death within 1 year of treatment. However, procedural difficulties and poor recruitment resulted in a decision to discontinue further clinical efforts in this trial.

Conclusions regarding the results of these initial clinical trials await further review and do not provide any conclusive data. However, as confirmed by the present consensus conference, CBAS can be used to treat extracranial carotid stenosis in selected subsets of patients with periprocedural complications that approach those reported for CEA. Nevertheless, a well-designed clinical trial is urgently required if we are to advise our patients about the efficacy of this new procedure.

III. CURRENT PRACTICE: TECHNICAL CONSIDERATIONS

Current practice suggests consideration be given to CBAS in several circumstances: anatomically high internal carotid stenoses, carotid restenosis following prior CEA, radiation-induced carotid stenosis, and occasional patients deemed high-risk due to severe medical comorbidities. These indications were considered and approved by this multidisciplinary consensus panel, and this represents a reasonable approach in view of the American Heart Association's position against use of CBAS for symptomatic carotid stenosis in NASCET-eligible patients until data are available from the planned clinical trial.

We have restricted our use of CBAS primarily to carotid restenosis after CEA (11). Symptomatic or asymptomatic carotid restenosis after CEA is relatively uncommon and is generally attributed to myointimal hyperplasia during the early postoperative period (within 36 months) or recurrent atherosclerosis thereafter (12–14). Surgical management of carotid restenosis is controversial for two major reasons. First, indications for operative management in the asymptomatic patient with high-grade (≥80%) restenosis remain controversial due to the low risk of stroke or progression to total occlusion (12,15). Second, reoperation is associated with an increased risk of perioperative neurological events and cranial nerve palsies (13,14). Because of these issues, some authors (16–18) recommend carotid angioplasty and stenting as an alternative to operative management.

We prospectively collected data and intervened using endovascular techniques on patients with symptomatic and asymptomatic (≥80%) carotid restenosis due to myointimal hyperplasia for the purpose of defining technical feasibility and periprocedural outcomes (11). Examples of pre- and postprocedural arteriograms (Fig. 1, 2) are presented and demonstrate placement of a 10 mm × 20 mm Wallstent (Boston Scientific Vascular, Natick, MA). A 4-mm low-profile balloon was used to initially dilate the lesions followed by placement of the Wallstent with poststent balloon dilatation to obtain the final result. Intravascular ultrasound was utilized to insure adequate apposition of the stent to the arterial wall. In these cases and all but one other case,

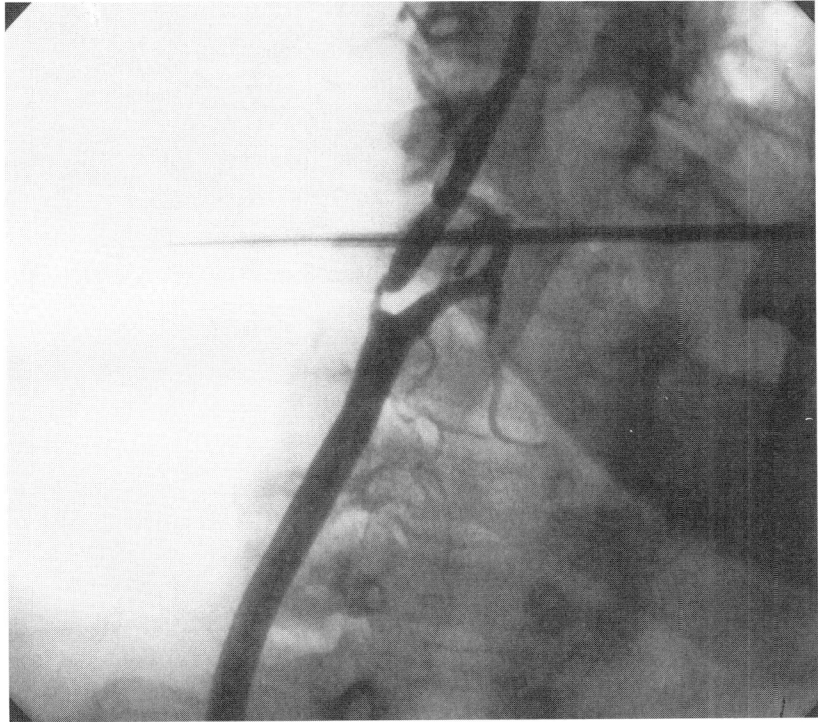

Figure 1 Preprocedural angiogram demonstrating a significant restenosis in a patient 22 months after prior CEA.

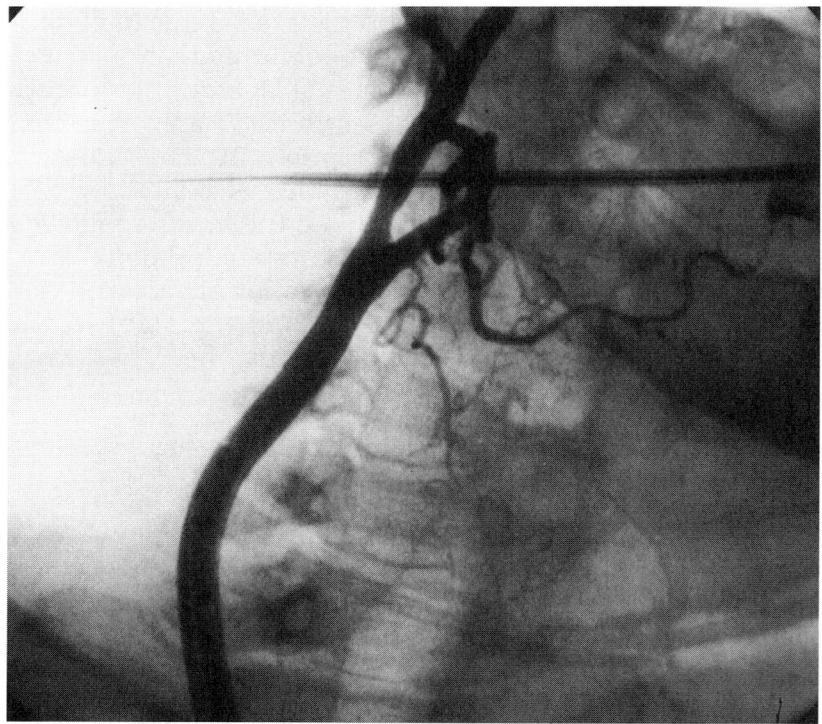

Figure 2 Angiographic result after CAS using a 10 × 20 Wall-stent.

stents were placed across the carotid bifurcation. Serial du-plex ultrasonography has demonstrated patency of all ex-ternal and internal carotid arteries.

In the originally treated group of 16 patients (17 proce-dures) (11), all procedures were completed technically. The series now has been expanded to 36 patients (39 proce-dures) in this category of restenosis. In-stent restenosis has been observed in four patients (10.2%). All remain asymp-tomatic. Two patients with in-stent restenosis (50–79%) are being followed clinically, while two other patients with high-grade restenosis ($\geq 80\%$) have been successfully treated with repeat balloon angioplasty alone. Although in-stent restenosis may be a significant problem in this group, management by repeat balloon angioplasty alone appears to be effective. However, longer-term follow-up will be necessary.

Based on our experience with the subset of restenosis patients as well as a review of results from retrospective analyses and one prospective clinical trial, these data suggest that an efficacy trial comparing the results of CEA and CBAS should proceed in this country. The CREST investigators have been funded to use a single stent in the trial; however, they anticipate use of run-in phase data and high-risk registry cases to introduce cerebral protection during the conduct of the trial.

IV. CREST ORGANIZATIONAL PLAN

The CREST investigators have received approval for funding from the NINDS (NIH) for a trial to compare the efficacy of CEA and CBAS in symptomatic patients with stenoses $\geq 50\%$. However, recognizing that CBAS is a relatively new procedure, each participating center will be required to complete a credentialing phase to reassure clinicians that the safety of these procedures has been reviewed and established before proceeding with the randomized phase of the trial.

Assuming that a credentialing phase that requires performance of up to 20 interventional procedures at each of 50 or more participating centers is completed to the satisfaction of the study's Interventional Management Committee, randomization of patients between the two treatments will then proceed. The primary outcome events for this clinical trial will include: 1) any stroke, myocardial infarction, or death during the 30-day perioperative or periprocedural period, or 2) ipsilateral stroke after 30 days. End-points will be reviewed by an Adjudication Committee blinded to the assigned treatment. Stroke will be determined by a positive TIA/stroke questionnaire confirmed by an evaluation by a neurologist. Myocardial infarction will be determined by ECG and enzyme abnormalities. Secondary goals include: 1) to describe differential efficacy of the two treatments in men and women, 2) to contrast perioperative-procedural (30-day) morbidity and postprocedural (after 30 days) mortality for CEA and CBAS, 3) to estimate and contrast the restenosis rates for the two procedures, 4) to identify subgroups of participants at differential risk for the two procedures, and 5) to evaluate differences in health-related quality-of-life issues and cost-effectiveness.

Differential efficacy assessment of CEA and CBAS based on gender is a secondary goal for CREST. In patients with high-grade asymptomatic stenosis reported by ACAS, CEA offered a 66% reduction in events over a 5-year period for men, but only a 17% reduction for women (5). In NASCET, while no differential gender effects were reported among symptomatic patients with stenosis greater than 70%, male patients demonstrated greater benefit after CEA than women for stenoses of 50–69% (19). While the causes for these examples of differential efficacy between genders are not well understood, the effect may be attributed to a higher complication rate for CEA in women, possibly caused by their reported smaller arterial sizes and a greater surgical morbidity. Unfortunately, neither ACAS nor NASCET suspected the possibility of a differential gender effect. However, given the results of these two randomized clinical trials, a requirement for a priori plans to evaluate the possibility of a differential gender effect has become an important component of CREST. Centers are being selected with a goal as high as 50% women in the randomized sample of patients and a minimum of 40% women.

Patients will be evaluated at baseline, 24-hr postprocedure, 30 days, 6, months, and thereafter at 6-month intervals. Baseline procedures will include a brief medical history and physical examination, a risk factor evaluation, performance of neurological status questionnaires, a neurological examination, ECG, and a baseline carotid duplex scan. The 30-day follow-up will include evaluation of the neurological status through questionnaires, ECG, and a follow-up carotid duplex scan. All 6-month follow-up visits will include a brief physical, completion of the neurological questionnaire, risk factor evaluation, and carotid duplex scan. All patients with a positive neurological status questionnaire will be evaluated by a neurologist. The sample size for the study is approximately 2500 symptomatic patients, which will be sufficient to detect a relative difference of 25–30% between treatment groups. Lesser differences would be considered sufficiently small to declare the treatments equivalent.

Opinions have varied about the participation of vascular surgeons in randomized clinical trials on carotid endarterectomy. While the value of our participation has been recommended (19), the emergence of clinical equipoise (16) between treatment groups as supported by a rigorous credentialing phase of CREST should reassure our colleagues about their participation as well as the ethical conduct of this trial.

V. CONCLUSIONS

Current clinical practice dictates that CBAS be considered in limited subsets of patients as outlined in this consensus document. Conduct of clinical trials (CREST and others) will provide Level I, II evidence upon which a firm clinical recommendation can be established. Until these data are available during the next several years, performance of CBAS should be limited to randomized clinical trials and defined unique subsets of high-risk patients. CEA continues to be recommended for management of most patients with symptomatic and asymptomatic extracranial carotid occlusive disease.

REFERENCES

1. North American Symptomatic Carotid Endarterectomy Trial Collaborators. Beneficial effect of carotid endarterectomy in symptomatic patients with high-grade carotid stenosis. N Engl J Med 1991; 325:445–453.
2. European Carotid Surgery Trialists' Collaborative Group. MCR European Carotid Surgery Trial: interim results for symptomatic patients with severe (70–99%) or with mild (0–29%) carotid stenosis. Lancet 1991; 337:1235–1243.
3. Mayberg MR, Wilson SE, Yatsu F, and the VA Symptomatic Carotid Stenosis Group. Carotid endarterectomy and prevention of cerebral ischemia in symptomatic carotid stenosis. JAMA 1991; 266:3289–3294.
4. Hobson RW, Weiss DG, Fields WS, Goldstone J, Moore WS, Towne JB, Wright CB, and the Veterans Affairs Cooperative Study Group. Efficacy of carotid endarterectomy for asymptomatic carotid stenosis. N Engl J Med 1993; 328:221–227.
5. Executive Committee for the Asymptomatic Carotid Atherosclerosis Study: endarterectomy for asymptomatic carotid stenosis. JAMA 1995; 273:1421–1428.
6. Freedman B. Equipoise and the ethics of clinical research. N Engl J Med 1987; 317:141–145.
7. Major ongoing stroke trials: carotid and vertebral artery transluminal angioplasty study (CAVATAS). Stroke 1996; 27:358.
8. Hobson RW, Brott T, Ferguson R, Roubin GS, Moore WS, Kuntz R, Howard G, Ferguson J. Letter to the Editor, Regarding "Statement regarding carotid angioplasty and stenting." J Vasc Surg 1997; 25:1117.
9. Naylor AR, Bolia A, Abbott RJ, et al. Randomized study of carotid angioplasty and stenting versus carotid endarterectomy. A stopped trial. J Vasc Surg 1998; 28:326–334.
10. Alberts MJ, McCann R, Smith TP, et al. A randomized trial: carotid stenting versus endarterectomy in patients with symptomatic carotid stenosis, study designs. J Neurovasc Dis 1997; Nov-Dec:228–234.
11. Hobson RW II, Goldstein JE, Jamil Z, Lee BC, Padberg FT Jr., Hanna AK, Gwertzman GA, Pappas PJ, Silva MB. Ca-

rotid restenosis: Operative and endovascular management. J Vasc Surg 1999; 29:228–238.

12. Lattimer CR, Burnand KG. Recurrent carotid stenosis after carotid endarterectomy. Br J Surg 1997; 84:1206–1219.
13. Stoney RJ, String ST. Recurrent carotid stenosis. Surgery 1976; 80(6):705–710.
14. Bartlett FF, Rapp JH, Goldstone J, Ehrenfeld WK, Stoney RJ. Recurrent carotid stenosis: operative strategy and late results. J Vasc Surg 1987; 5:452–456.
15. Healy DA, Zierler RE, Nicholls SC, Clowes AW, Primozich JF, Bergelin RO, Strandness DE Jr. Long-term follow-up and clinical outcome of carotid restenosis. J Vasc Surg 1989; 10: 662–669.
16. Bergeron P, Chambran P, Benichou H, Alessandri C. Recurrent carotid disease: will stents be an alternative to surgery? J Endovasc Surg 1996; 3:76–79.
17. Yadav JS, Roubin GS, King P, Iyer S, Vitek J. Angioplasty and stenting for restenosis after carotid endarterectomy. Initial experience. Stroke 1996; 27:2075–2079.
18. Theron J, Raymond J, Casasco A, Courtheoux F. Percutaneous angioplasty of atherosclerotic and postsurgical stenosis of carotid arteries. Am J Neurorad 1987; 8:495–500.
19. Barnett HJM, Taylor DW, Eliasziw M, Fox AJ, Ferguson GG, Haynes RB, Rankin RN, Clagett GP, Hachinski VC, Sackett DL, Thorpe KE, Meldrum HE, for the North American Symptomatic Carotid Endarterectomy Trial Collaborators. Benefit of carotid endarterectomy in patients with symptomatic moderate or severe stenosis. N Engl J Med 1998; 339:1415–1425.

10
Patient Selection, Complications, and Periprocedural Considerations in Carotid Artery Stenting

Richard D. Fessler
Wayne State University, Detroit, Michigan

Adnan I. Qureshi, Andrew J. Ringer, Lee R. Guterman, and L. Nelson Hopkins
State University of New York at Buffalo, Buffalo, New York

I. INTRODUCTION

Extracranial carotid surgery continues to evolve and evoke debate. Since the first surgical reconstruction of the carotid artery in 1951 by Carrea et al., issues regarding proper technique, patient selection, timing of surgery, and the utility of surgical versus medical therapy have been debated (1,2). The current medical literature supports the role of carotid endarterectomy (CEA) on the basis of several prospective randomized clinical trials. The results of the North American Symptomatic Carotid Endarterectomy Trial (NASCET), the Asymptomatic Carotid Atherosclerosis Study (ACAS), and the European Carotid Surgery Trial (ECST) have proven the efficacy and durability of this operation in patients with carotid stenosis (3–5). Patients benefiting include those with greater than 70% stenosis documented by angiography and recent nondisabling stroke, hemispheric transient ischemic attacks (TIAs), or amaurosis fugax. Symptomatic and asymptomatic stenoses of 60% or more, in men, show a reduced 5-year stroke rate if surgical morbidity and mortality are low (4,6). The recent introduction of carotid artery stenting (CAS) has added another therapeutic technique to the extracranial carotid revascularization debate.

In the coronary and peripheral circulations, endoluminal angioplasty and stenting has become established as a routine procedure. Since the first description of endoluminal angioplasty by Gruntzig and Hopff, improved technical expertise and technological advances in endovascular surgery have resulted in widespread application of endoluminal techniques (7). In many cases of coronary and renal artery disease, endoluminal techniques have supplanted traditional open surgical approaches. The effectiveness of angioplasty and stenting has been proven by prospective trials in many cases. The BENESTENT trial compared coronary angioplasty with balloon-expandable stenting of coro-

nary atherosclerotic lesions and proved that both procedures were safe and effective (8). By contrast, early
experience with angioplasty in the extracranial and intracranial circulation was associated with significant morbidity. Reserved for seriously ill, symptomatic patients, the
procedure was associated with complication rates ranging
from 12 to 33% (9–11). However, a recent report suggests
that improved pharmacological management and the ability to deliver microcatheters and balloons into the extracranial and intracranial vasculature with greater ease have
significantly lessened the risk of intracranial angioplasty
(12). Similar to the early experience with intracranial angioplasty, initial reports of carotid angioplasty and stenting
have emphasized patients considered to be at higher risk
for complication with CEA (13–18).

II. PATIENT SELECTION IN CAS

The results of NASCET (3) suggest that the standard for an-
gioplasty-assisted CAS in symptomatic patients should be
a combined morbidity and mortality of less than 6%. Several points germane to patient selection and outcome in
NASCET bear particular relevance to CAS. NASCET was
subject to significant selection bias in patient enrollment
and surgical expertise. During the NASCET enrollment period, the mortality rate for Medicare beneficiaries undergoing CEA was 3% versus 0.6% in NASCET enrollees undergoing CEA (19). In addition, the surgical results obtained
by NASCET and ACAS surgeons are often not duplicated in
the community. Surgical results typically are better at
high-volume centers such as study sites (20,21). It should
be noted that surgeons tend to self-report lower rates of
complication than independent observers, and community
complication rates for CEA are often higher than the morbidity and mortality rates reported in NASCET and ACAS.

Hartmann et al. reported an 8.3% rate of stroke or death within 30 days with twice as many symptomatic as asymptomatic patients affected (22). Elevated surgical perioperative risk may negate the benefits of the procedure (23,24). It has been estimated that for every 2% increase in the perioperative CEA complication rate, the 5-year benefit decreases by approximately 20% (25). Additional evidence for selection bias can be inferred from the Carotid and Vertebral Artery Transluminal Angioplasty Study (CAVATAS) in which patients were prospectively randomized to CEA or carotid angioplasty. The morbidity and mortality for each treatment group was approximately 10%, with no statistically significant benefit derived from either procedure relative to the other (M. Brown, Transcatheter Cardiovascular Therapeutics, The Eleventh Annual Symposium, Washington, DC, September 1999).

The Global Carotid Artery Stent Registry contains data on 4865 cervical carotid artery stent procedures performed in 33 centers with ongoing data collection. Recent results were reported on data accrued from 1997 to 1999 (26). The combined (perioperative 30 day) major and minor stroke rate and procedure-related death rate was 4.77%. The minor and major stroke rates were 2.45% and 1.48%, respectively (minor stroke is defined as a neurological deficit that resolves within 1 week, and deficits persisting beyond 1 week are classified as major stroke). The mortality rate was 0.84%. The periprocedural transient ischemic attack (TIA) rate was 2.45%. Interestingly, over the course of compilation of the registry, the overall complication rate has diminished. A learning curve of approximately 50 cases was noted with centers performing fewer than 50 cases having significantly higher rates of major and minor strokes than those performing more than 50 cases (26). The registry suggests that complication rates associated with CAS approximate those of CEA.

Although it is unlikely that CAS can supplant CEA in

"NASCET-eligible" patients in the near future, the relative role of CEA and CAS is undetermined for several significant subgroups of patients who are at increased risk for stroke or death with CEA. Patients with contralateral carotid artery occlusion documented by angiography, an ischemic lesion ipsilateral to the stenosed carotid artery, elevated diastolic blood pressure (>90 mmHg), or diabetes mellitus may have double the risk of stroke or death with CEA (6). Mericle et al. reported excellent results with CAS in patients with contralateral occlusion, suggesting that CAS is a viable treatment option in this patient population (16). Other risk factors for CEA include recent stroke, crescendo TIAs, stroke in evolution, contralateral hypoglossal or recurrent laryngeal nerve palsy, congestive heart failure, age greater than 75 years, combined CEA and coronary surgery, unstable angina, renal failure, recurrent stenosis, and radiation-induced stenosis. Lanzino et al. reported a series of 21 patients treated by stenting for recurrent carotid artery stenosis following CEA (14) (Figs. 1 and 2). The overall rate of combined major and minor stroke or death was 0%. There were no cardiac complications. One patient had a periprocedural TIA. Lopes et al. reported 20 patients with unstable cardiac status who underwent CAS prior to CABG (15). One patient suffered a transient neurological deficit (TIA); one patient developed an asymptomatic subendocardial myocardial infarction (MI); and one patient suffered a groin hematoma. This experience is in contradistinction to the CEA guidelines published by the American Heart Association in which the incidence of stroke, MI, and death is 16.44% for combined CEA and CABG, 26.15% for CEA followed by CABG, and 16.35% for CABG followed by CEA (27). Angiographic risk factors include long, irregular plaques, the aforementioned contralateral carotid artery occlusion, tandem stenosis, intraluminal thrombus, and high cervical bifurcation stenosis (28).

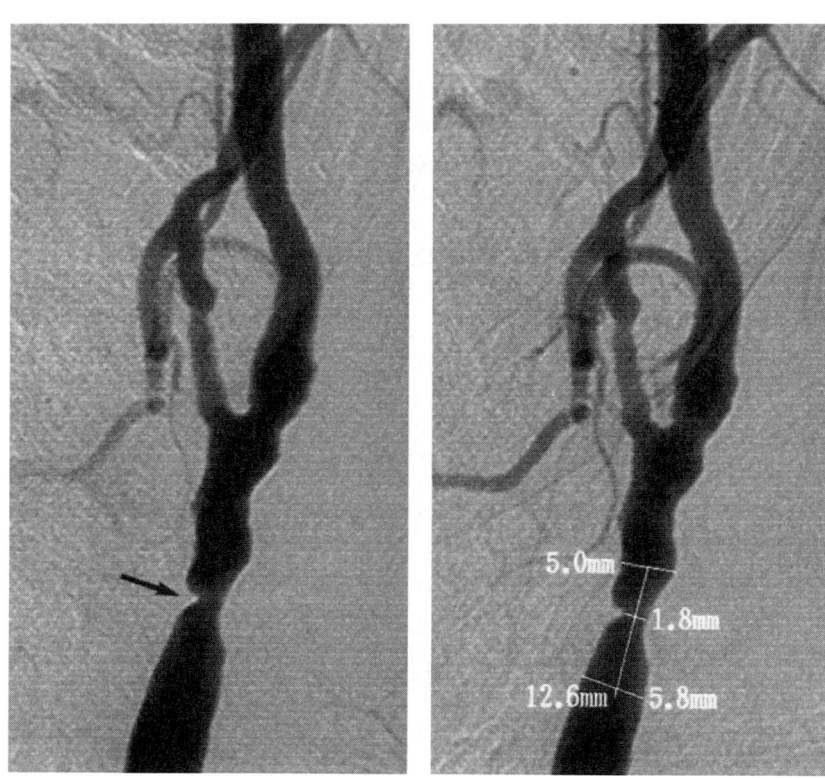

Figure 1 The patient presented with symptomatic carotid artery restenosis following previous carotid endarterectomy. Left common carotid artery injection, lateral views, before stenting. (Left) Arrow denotes region of stenosis. (Right) Measurements are shown.

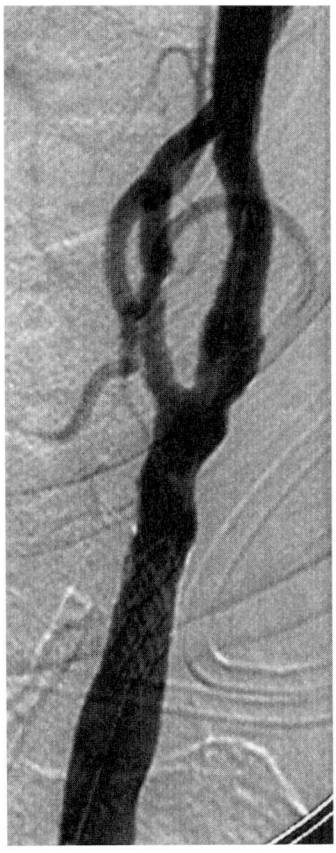

Figure 2 Final angiographic result following carotid artery stenting. A stent has been placed across the stenotic region. The patient was discharged to home in good condition 1 day following stent placement.

III. RISKS OF CAS

Many risks inherent to CEA are obviated in CAS. All issues related to surgical dissection, i.e., high cervical bifurcation, contralateral cranial nerve palsies, recurrent stenosis, are obviated during CAS. As discussed previously, CAS may be equal or superior to CEA in some patient subgroups (14–18,29). However, increased periprocedural risk occurs for both CEA and CAS in those patients with unstable neurological status, congestive heart failure, unstable angina, intraluminal thrombus, and long, irregular lesions. Several risks are germane to CAS. Access-related complications occur in as many as 2% of patients (30). The risk of periprocedural emboli is higher for CAS than CEA. Transcranial Doppler ultrasound studies have documented an increased rate of high-intensity transient signals in patients with severe carotid stenosis (31,32). These signals are believed to represent microemboli emanating from regions of arterial narrowing in which alterations in blood flow favor the formation of thrombi. Angioplasty of such lesions in the absence of distal protection may release a significant "microembolic load" that is predominantly deposited in the distal watershed zones (33).

Ohki et al., using explanted human carotid artery plaques, have shown that all carotid plaques release embolic particles during angioplasty and stenting procedures (34). The mean number of particles released appears to relate to the occurrence of perioperative complications in both CEA and CAS. In 105 patients undergoing 112 procedures, Jordan et al. noted that patients with neurological complications had an average of 56.8 microemboli documented by periprocedural Doppler whereas those without neurological complications averaged 31.2 microemboli ($p <$ 0.02) (35). Similar findings have been documented during CEA in which the absolute number of microemboli detected by Doppler ultrasonography correlated with perioperative neurological events (36,37).

Emboli are typically liberated during periods of vessel and plaque manipulation. Thus, maneuvers such as guidewire placement, pre- and postdeployment balloon angioplasty, and stent deployment are associated with liberation of microemboli (38). The vast majority of periprocedural stent complications are related to emboli. McCleary et al. reported showers of emboli in association with guidewire manipulation and even more so with balloon deflation following angioplasty (39). However, it should be noted that this group did not utilize preprocedure antiplatelet therapy, and the experience level of the neurointerventionist is unknown. Independent risk factors for periprocedural stroke during CAS include echolucent plaques, long angiographic lesions, contralateral occlusion, and stenosis greater than 90% (34,40).

IV. DISTAL PROTECTION

Currently, in the absence of distal protection devices, it is unlikely that CAS will supplant CEA for patients who present as "NASCET-eligible." Several distal protection devices will become available in the near future. Those likely to be most successful rely on a low-profile balloon or "filter" that can be passed through the lesion and deployed distally. In this technique, the balloon or filter is mounted on the distal end of a guidewire, and the balloon is inflated or the filter opened in the native carotid lumen distal to the target lesion. With the balloon technique, embolic debris is either flushed into the external carotid artery (ECA) circulation or aspirated into a catheter with associated flushing. Filters trap debris and collapse when pulled back into the guidecatheter. The distal protection technique was first described by Theron et al., who used a triple coaxial catheter with a latex balloon mounted at the distal end (41). Debris is flushed and aspirated after stent deployment. Using this technique, TIA rates as low as 0.9% and stroke rates as low as 1.6% have been reported (38).

V. ANTIPLATELET THERAPY

Several factors predispose patients to thromboembolic events during CAS. Carotid artery angioplasty and stent placement results in denuded, damaged endothelium, which is highly thrombogenic. In addition, the stents and catheters are themselves thrombogenic (42–44). Platelet aggregation over a damaged endothelial surface is associated with an increased risk of thromboembolic complications including stent occlusion and distal stroke. Platelet adhesion is initiated upon exposure of the subendothelium secondary to wire or catheter manipulation or during angioplasty and stent placement (45,46). Platelet adhesion results in secondary activation of membrane glycoprotein (GP) IIb/IIIa receptors, which subsequently bind fibrinogen and initiate further platelet aggregation through amplification mediated by release of platelet adenosine diphosphate, thromboxane A2, and serotonin. Abciximab, a recently FDA-approved antiplatelet agent consisting of a murine monoclonal antibody to the GP IIb/IIIa receptor, inhibits the adhesion of fibrinogen to platelets by blocking the GP IIb/IIIa site (47,48). Thus, platelet-mediated thrombus propagation can be blocked.

Current studies of abciximab use during stenting of extracranial carotid artery disease are lacking. However, based on extensive study in the coronary literature, the use of oral antiplatelet agents before and after stent placement has become routine (49–52). The Ticlopidine Aspirin Stent Evaluation Study (TASTE) assessed the efficacy of combination aspirin and ticlopidine therapy in patients undergoing elective or bailout coronary stenting and showed excellent short-term outcomes (49). The Multicenter Aspirin and Ticlopidine Trial After Intracoronary Stenting (MATTIS) showed a strong trend toward diminished adverse outcomes in patients treated with aspirin and ticlopidine versus aspirin plus warfarin after coronary stenting, with a significant decline in adverse bleeding outcomes (50). The Evaluation of Platelet IIb/IIIa Inhibitor for Stenting (EPISTENT) Trial showed that both percutaneous transluminal coronary angioplasty (PTCA) and stenting are safer with abciximab (52). The Evaluation of 7E3 for Prevention of Ischemic Complications (EPIC) Trial showed that ischemic complications of PTCA were reduced with abciximab, although bleeding complications were slightly increased (53). Our preliminary experience with abciximab in high-risk CAS patients suggests that it is safe and procedures can be performed with minimal morbidity (A. I. Qureshi et al., personal communication). Elective CAS at our institution is typically performed following preoperative administration of aspirin and ticlopidine or clopidogrel. At present, symptomatic and asymptomatic patients with long, irregular lesions are prophylactically treated with abciximab based on a retrospective analysis of our patient data (A. I. Qureshi et al., personal communication).

VI. TECHNICAL CONSIDERATIONS IN CAS

A. Perioperative Antiplatelet Therapy

Although the general technique involved in CAS is straightforward, several points are worth emphasizing. Perioperative administration of antiplatelet agents (as previously discussed) has been shown to diminish the occurrence of thromboembolic complications. The use of aspirin (325 mg) and ticlopidine (250 mg twice daily) or clopidogrel (75 mg daily) for 48–72 h before the procedure and for approximately 4 weeks after the procedure is based on the extensive experience in the coronary vasculature (54,55). The Clopidogrel Versus Aspirin in Patients at Risk of Ischaemic Events (CAPRIE) study demonstrated an 8–10% relative risk reduction of ischemic stroke, MI, or vascular deaths in patients taking 75 mg of clopidogrel daily. In addition, patients exhibited improved tolerance relative to ticlopidine (56).

In those patients presenting for nonelective stent procedures or those considered high risk for thromboembolic complication, a single oral loading dose of clopidogrel (450 mg) followed by intraprocedural use of intravenous abciximab (0.25 mg/kg bolus followed by 10 µg/kg/min for 12 h) is utilized along with partial heparinization. To avoid significant bleeding complications with GP IIb/IIIa antagonists, partial heparinization is important. Heparin is administered to maintain an activated coagulation time (ACT) of approximately 200–250 sec (<200 sec post procedure) (57). Bleeding complications with abciximab have been minor in our experience (A. I. Qureshi et al., personal communication). However, concerns exist regarding the inability to reverse the effects of abciximab acutely without platelet transfusion. Newer agents may soon become available that will obviate some of these concerns (58).

B. Catheter Management

Accessing the common carotid artery proximal to the bifurcation with the guide catheter can occasionally be difficult secondary to tortuosity of the aortic arch or brachiocephalic vessels. The importance of minimizing trauma to the vessels cannot be overemphasized for prevention of release of thromboemboli. Before advancing catheters into the common carotid artery (CCA), we have achieved our target ACT and have administered a GP IIb/IIIa antagonist in those patients considered high risk. A diagnostic catheter attached to heparinized flush (5 U/ml) is passed into the CCA. After obtaining a road map, we advance a 0.035-in. glidewire into the ECA. Care is taken to avoid torquing the wire against the plaque, rotating the wire within the ECA, or moving the distal wire tip to and fro within the distal ECA. Following wire placement in the distal ECA, the diagnostic catheter is advanced into the ECA after which the glidewire is removed and exchanged with a superstiff 0.035-in. Amplatz wire (Boston Scientific, Natick, MA). Although the exchange can be performed with one less step by passing the Amplatz wire directly into the ECA without first passing the glidewire and diagnostic catheter, the Amplatz wire is difficult to maneuver and can cause intimal damage at the level of the bifurcation or elsewhere during attempted manipulation into the ECA. Torquing or buckling of the Amplatz wire against a highly stenotic bifurcation lesion can result in release of thromboemboli or, in some cases, in occlusion of the internal carotid artery Similarly, when advancing guidecatheters into the CCA, it is important to maintain constant tension on the exchange wire to avoid distal perforation of the ECA or buckling against the CCA bifurcation. Guidecatheters are continuously flushed with heparinized saline.

In some patients, the tortuous origin of the supraaortic vessels makes passage of the guidecatheter difficult, even with a stable superstiff exchange wire in the ECA. Any resistance encountered during passage of the guidecatheter from the aortic arch to the CCA should be evaluated. The stiff portion of the Amplatz wire often significantly alters the brachiocephalic-CCA junction relative to its native position. Asking the patient to inhale and hold his or her breath will stretch the origins of the great vessels and often provide enough straightening of the vessel origins to allow passage of the guidecatheter into the CCA.

C. CAS and Periprocedural Hemodynamic Instability

The occurrence of hemodynamic instability following CEA is a well-recognized event and may include hypertension, hypotension, or bradycardia (59–61). Procedure-related hemodynamic instability occurs in as many as 70% of patients undergoing CAS (17,62). Qureshi et al. observed hypertension in 38.8%, bradycardia in 27.5%, and hypotension in 22.4% of patients in the periprocedural period, many of whom required vasopressors for a sustained length of time (40). Intraprocedural hypotension was the greatest predictor of postprocedural hypotension, although postprocedural hypotension did occur in the absence of intraprocedural hypotension and was associated with a history of previous MI. Intraprocedural hypotension and bradycardia are managed with a combination of atropine, dopamine, and/or aramine as necessary. Pressors are generally weaned over 6–18 hr in an intensive-care-unit setting.

VII. CONCLUSIONS

Several patient subgroups may benefit from CAS (Table 1). Patients for whom CEA poses a significantly increased risk for complication include those with contralateral carotid artery occlusion, severe tandem stenosis ipsilateral to the stenosed carotid artery, elevated diastolic blood pressure (>90 mmHg), or diabetes mellitus (6). Additional patients who should be considered candidates for CAS include those with recurrent stenosis, patients with carotid stenosis who are pre-CABG, those with high carotid bifurcations, recurrent stenosis, contralateral cranial nerve palsies, radiation-induced stenosis, severe medical comorbidities, and tandem lesions. Although the current indications for CAS are not well defined, it appears that CAS compares favorably to CEA in high-risk surgical patients and in centers having low surgical volumes. Patients meeting NASCET and ACAS inclusion criteria represent a select patient group that should not be considered for CAS as an initial intervention according to the results from the Carotid Stent Registry (26) and large case series.

The role of periprocedural pharmacologic management

Table 1 High-Risk Patients Who May
Benefit from CAS

Medical
  Pre-CABG
  Unstable angina
  Congestive heart failure
  Uncontrolled hypertension
  Multiple medical comorbidities
Angiographic
  Tandem lesions
  Contralateral carotid occlusion
Surgical
  Recurrent carotid artery stenosis
  Radiation-associated stenosis
  High cervical bifurcation
  Low cervical bifurcation
  Morbid obesity
Neurological
  Recurrent symptoms on anticoagulation
  High risk for CAS *and* CEA

cannot be overemphasized. Antiplatelet agents confer significant benefit in the periprocedural period. The role of GP IIb/IIIa antagonists remains to be conclusively determined, but initial experience in the coronary circulation and in anecdotal reports may support its use in high-risk patients undergoing CAS. Distal protection devices in conjunction with antiplatelet agents may significantly reduce the occurrence of periprocedural embolic phenomena, which are currently the most feared complication of CAS.

ACKNOWLEDGMENT

We thank Paul H. Dressel for preparation of the illustrations.

REFERENCES

1. Carrea R, Molins M, Murphy G. Surgical treatment of spontaneous thrombosis of the internal carotid artery in the neck: carotid-carotidal anastomosis: report of a case. Acta Neurol Latinoamer 1951; 1:71–78.
2. Robertson JT. Carotid endarterectomy: a saga of clinical science, personalities, and evolving technology. The Willis lecture. Stroke 1997; 29:2563–2567.
3. North American Symptomatic Carotid Endarterectomy Trial Collaborators. Beneficial effect of carotid endarterectomy in symptomatic patients with high-grade stenosis. N Engl J Med 1991; 325:445–453.
4. The Asymptomatic Carotid Atherosclerosis Study Group. Endarterectomy for asymptomatic carotid artery stenosis. JAMA 1995; 273:1421–1428.
5. European Carotid Surgery Trialists' Collaborative Group: MRC European Carotid Surgery Trial. Interim results for asymptomatic patients with severe (70–99%) or with mild (0–29%) carotid stenosis. Lancet 1991; 337:1235–1241.
6. Barnett HJM, Taylor DW, Eliasziw M, Fox AJ, Ferguson GG, Haynes RB, Rankin RN, Clagett GP, Hachinski VC, Sackett DL, Thorpe KE, Meldrum HE, for the North American Symptomatic Carotid Endarterectomy Trial Collaborators. Benefit of carotid endarterectomy in patients with symptomatic moderate or severe stenosis. N Engl J Med 1998; 339:1415–1425.
7. Gruntzig A, Hopff H. Percutaneous recanalization after chronic arterial occlusion with a new dilator-catheter. J Dtsch Med Wochenschr 1974; 99:2502–2510.
8. Serruys PW, De Jaegere P, Kiemeneij F, Macaya C, Rutsch W, Heyndrickx G, Emanuelsson H, Marco J, Legrand V, Materne P, Belardi J, Sigwart U, Colombo A, Goy JJ, van der Heuvel, Delcan J, Morel M. A comparison of balloon-expandable-stent implantation with balloon angioplasty in patients with coronary artery disease. The BENESTENT Study Group. N Engl J Med 1994; 331:489–495.
9. Clark WM, Barnwell SL, Nesbit G, O'Neill OR, Wynn ML, Coull BM. Safety and efficacy of percutaneous transluminal

angioplasty for intracranial atherosclerotic stenosis. Stroke 1995; 26:1200–1204.

10. Higashida RT, Tsai FY, Halbach VV, Dowd CF, Hieshima GB. Cerebral percutaneous transluminal angioplasty. Heart Dis Stroke 1993; 2:497–502.

11. Terada T, Higashida RT, Halbach VV, Dowd CF, Nakai E, Yokote H, Itakura T, Hieshima GB. Transluminal angioplasty for arteriosclerotic disease of the distal vertebral and basilar arteries. J Neurol Neurosurg Psychiatry 1996; 60: 377–381.

12. Connors JJ 3rd, Wojak JC. Percutaneous transluminal angioplasty for intracranial atherosclerotic lesions: evolution of technique and short-term results. J Neurosurg 1999; 91: 415–423.

13. Diethrich EB, Ndiaye M, Reid DB. Stenting in the carotid artery: initial experience in 110 patients. J Endovasc Surg 1996; 3:42–62.

14. Lanzino G, Mericle RA, Lopes DK, Wakhloo AK, Guterman LR, Hopkins LN. Percutaneous transluminal angioplasty and stent placement for recurrent carotid artery stenosis. J Neurosurg 1999; 90:688–794.

15. Lopes DK, Mericle RA, Lanzino G, Wakhloo AK, Guterman LR, Hopkins LN. Carotid angioplasty and stenting before coronary artery bypass grafting (abstr). Neurosurgery 1998; 43:686.

16. Mericle RA, Kim S, Lanzino G, Lopes DK, Wakhloo AK, Guterman LR, Hopkins LN. Carotid artery angioplasty and use of stents in high-risk patients with contralateral occlusions. J Neurosurg 1999; 90:1031–1036.

17. Yadav JS, Roubin GS, Iyer S, Vitek J, King P, Jordan WD, Fisher WS. Elective stenting of the extracranial arteries. Circulation 1997; 95:376–381.

18. Yadav JS, Roubin GS, King P, Iyer S, Vitek J. Angioplasty and stenting for restenosis after carotid endarterectomy. Initial experience. Stroke 1996; 27:2075–2079.

19. Hsai DC, Krushat M, Mmosoe LM. Epidemiology of carotid endarterectomies among Medicare beneficiaries. J Vasc Surg 1992; 16:201–208.

20. Barnett HJM, Eliasziw M, Meldrum HE, Taylor DW. Do the facts and figures warrant a 10-fold increase in the perfor-

mance of carotid endarterectomy on asymptomatic patients? Neurology 1996; 46:603–608.

21. Perry JR, Szalai JP, Norris JW, for the Canadian Stroke Consortium. Consensus against both endarterectomy and routine screening for asymptomatic carotid artery stenosis. Arch Neurol 1997; 54:25–28.

22. Hartmann A, Hupp T, Koch HC, Dollinger P, Stapf C, Schmidt R, Hofmeister C, Thompson JL, Marx P, Mast H. Prospective study on the complication rate of carotid surgery. Cerebrovasc Dis 1999; 9:152–156.

23. Stukenborg GJ. Comparison of carotid endarterectomy outcomes from randomized controlled trials and Medicare administrative data bases. Arch Neurol 1997; 54:826–832.

24. Hannan EL, Popp AJ, Tranmer B, Fuestel P, Waldman J, Shah D. Relationship between provider volume and mortality for carotid endarterectomy in New York State. Stroke 1998; 29:2292–2297.

25. Chassin MR. Appropriate use of carotid endarterectomy. N Engl J Med 1998; 339:1468–1471.

26. Wholey MH. Global Carotid Artery Stent Registry: updated results. Carotid Intervention 1999; 1:94–96.

27. Moore WS, Barnett HJM, Beebe HG, Bernstein EF, Brener BJ, Brott T, Caplan LR, Day A, Goldstone J, Hobson RW II, Kempczinski RF, Matchar DB, Mayberg MR, Nicolaides AN, Norris JW, Ricotta JJ, Robertson JT, Rutherford RB, Thomas D, Toole JF, Trout HH III, Wiebers DO. Guidelines for Carotid Endarterectomy. A multidisciplinary consensus statement from the Ad Hoc Committee, American Heart Association. Stroke 1995; 26:188–201.

28. Lanzino G, Fessler RD, Mericle RA, Wakhloo AK, Guterman LR, Hopkins LN. Angioplasty and stenting for carotid artery stenosis: indications, techniques, results, and complications. Neurosurgery Quarterly 2000; 10:83–99.

29. Mathur A, Roubin GS, Iyer SS, Piamsonboon C, Liu MW, Gomez CR, Yadav JS, Chastain HD, Fox LM, Dean LS, Vitek JJ. Predictors of stroke complicating carotid artery stenting. Circulation 1998; 97:1239–1245.

30. Kiemeneij F, Laarman GJ, Odekerken D, Slagboom T, van der Wieken R. A randomized comparison of percutaneous transluminal coronary angioplasty by radial, brachial, and

femoral approaches: the access study. J Am Coll Cardiol 1997; 29:1269–1275.

31. Ries S, Schminke U, Daffertshofer M, Hennerici M. High-intensity transcranial signals in carotid artery disease. Cerebrovasc Dis 1995; 5:124–127.

32. Siebler M, Sitzer M, Rose G, Bendfeldt D, Steinmetz H. Silent cerebral embolism caused by neurologically symptomatic high-grade carotid stenosis: event rates before and after carotid endarterectomy. Brain 1993; 116:1005–1015.

33. Fessler RD, Lanzino G, Guterman LR, Miletich RS, Lopes DK, Hopkins LN. Improved cerebral perfusion after stenting of a petrous carotid stenosis: technical case report. Neurosurgery 1999; 45:638–642.

34. Ohki T, Marin ML, Lyon RT, Berdejo GI, Soundararajan K, Ohki M, Yuan JG, Faries PL, Wain RA, Sanchez LA, Suggs WD, Veith FJ. Ex vivo human carotid artery bifurcation stenting: correlation of lesion characteristics with embolic potential. J Vasc Surg 1998; 27:463–471.

35. Jordan WD Jr, Voellinger DC, Doblar DD, Plyushcheva NP, Fisher WS, McDowell HA. Microemboli detected by transcranial Doppler monitoring in patients during carotid angioplasty versus carotid endarterectomy. Cardiovasc Surg 1997; 7:33–38.

36. Ackerstaff RG, Jansen C, Moll FL, Vermeulen FE, Hamerlijnck RP, Mauser HW. The significance of microemboli detection by means of transcranial Doppler ultrasonography monitoring in carotid endarterectomy. J Vasc Surg 1995; 21:963–969.

37. Jansen C, Ramos LM, van Heesewijk JP, Moll FL, van Gijn J, Ackerstaff RG. Impact of microembolism and hemodynamic changes in the brain during carotid endarterectomy. Stroke 1994; 25:992–997.

38. Henry M, Amor M, Henry I, Frid N, Hugel M. Cerebral protection and carotid angioplasty. Carotid Intervention 1999; 1: 66–75.

39. McCleary AJ, Nelson M, Dearden NM, Calvey TAJ, Gough MJ. Cerebral haemodynamics and embolization during carotid angioplasty in high-risk patients. Br J Surg 1998; 85: 771–774.

40. Qureshi AI, Luft AR, Sharma M, Janardhan V, Lopes DK, Khan J, Guterman LR, Hopkins LN. Frequency and determinants of postprocedural hemodynamic instability after carotid angioplasty and stenting. Stroke 1999; 30: 2086–2093.

41. Theron J, Courtheoux P, Alachkar F, Bouvard G, Maiza D. New triple coaxial catheter system for carotid angioplasty with cerebral protection. Am J Neuroradiol 1990; 11:869–874.

42. Bourassa MG, Cantin M, Sandborn EB, Pederson E. Scanning electron microscopy of surface irregularities and thrombogenesis of polyurethane and polyethylene coronary catheters. Circulation 1976; 53:992–996.

43. Anderson JH, Bianturco C, Wallace S, Dodd GD. A scanning electron microscopic study of angiographic catheters and guide wires. Radiology 1974; 111:567–571.

44. Krupski WC, Bass A, Kelly AB, Marzec UM, Hanson SR, Harker LA. Heparin-resistant thrombus formation by endovascular stents in baboons. Circulation 1990; 82:570–577.

45. Hynes RO. Integrins: a family of cell surface receptors. Cell 1987; 48:549–554.

46. Smyth SS, Joneckis CC, Parise LV. Regulation of vascular integrins. Blood 1993; 81:2827–2843.

47. Coller BS, Peerschke EI, Scudder LE, Sullivan CA. A murine monoclonal antibody that completely blocks the binding of fibrinogen to platelets produces a thrombasthenic-like state in normal platelets and binds to glycoproteins IIb and/or IIIa. J Clin Invest 1983; 72:325–338.

48. Coller BS, Scudder LE, Beer J, Gold HK, Folts JD, Cavagnaro J, Jordan R, Wagner C, Iuliucci J, Knight D. Monoclonal antibodies to platelet glycoprotein IIb/IIIa as antithrombotic agents. Ann NY Acad Sci 1991; 614:193–213.

49. Goods CM, al-Shaibi KF, Liu MW, Yadav JS, Mathur A, Jain SP, Dean LS, Iyer SS, Parks JM, Roubin GS. Comparison of aspirin alone versus aspirin plus ticlopidine after coronary artery stenting. Am J Cardiol 1996; 78:1042–1044.

50. Urban P, Macaya C, Rupprecht HJ, Kiemeneij F, Emanuelsson H, Fontanelli A, Pieper M, Wesseling T, Sagnard L. Randomized evaluation of anticoagulation versus antiplate-

let therapy after coronary stent implantation in high-risk patients: the multicenter aspirin and ticlopidine trial after intracoronary stenting (MATTIS). Circulation 1998; 98:2126–2132.

51. Bertrand ME, Legrand V, Boland J, Fleck E, Bonnier J, Emmanuelson H, Brolix M, Missalt L, Chierchia S, Casaccia M, Niccoli L, Oto A, White C, Webb-Peploe M, Van Belle E, McFadden EP. Randomized multicenter comparison of conventional anticoagulation versus antiplatelet therapy in unplanned and elective coronary stenting. The full anticoagulation versus aspirin and ticlopidine (FANTASTIC) study. Circulation 1998; 98:1597–1603.

52. The EPISTENT Investigators. Randomised placebo-controlled and balloon-angioplasty-controlled trial to assess safety of coronary stenting with use of platelet glycoprotein-IIb/IIIa blockade. Evaluation of Platelet IIb/IIIa Inhibitor for Stenting. Lancet 1998; 352:87–92.

53. The EPIC Investigators. Use of a monoclonal antibody directed against the platelet glycoprotein IIb/IIIa receptor in high-risk coronary angioplasty. N Engl J Med 1994; 330: 956–961.

54. Gregorini L, Marco J, Fajadet J, Bernies M, Cassagneau B, Brunel P, Bossi IM, Mannucci PM. Ticlopidine and aspirin pretreatment reduces coagulation and platelet activation during coronary dilatation procedures. J Am Coll Cardiol 1997; 29:13–20.

55. Colombo A, Hall P, Nakamura S, Almagor Y, Maiello L, Martini G, Gaglione A, Goldberg SL, Tobis JM. Intracoronary stenting without anticoagulation accomplished with intravascular ultrasound guidance. Circulation 1995; 91:1676–1688.

56. CAPRIE Steering Committee. A randomised, blinded, trial of clopidogrel versus aspirin in patients at risk of ischaemic events (CAPRIE). Lancet 1996; 348:1329–1339.

57. The EPILOG Investigators. Platelet glycoprotein IIb/IIIa receptor blockade and low-dose heparin during percutaneous coronary revascularization. N Engl J Med 1997; 336:1689–1696.

58. Randomised placebo-controlled trial of effect of eptifibatide on complications of percutaneous coronary intervention:

IMPACT-II. Integrilin to Minimise Platelet Aggregation and Coronary Thrombosis-II. Lancet 1997; 349:1422–1428.

59. Bove EL, Fry WJ, Gross WS, Stanley JC. Hypotension and hypertension as consequences of baroreceptor dysfunction following carotid endarterectomy. Surgery 1979; 85:633–637.
60. Hans SS, Glover JL. The relationship of cardiac and neurological complications to blood pressure changes following carotid endarterectomy. Am Surg 1995; 61:356–359.
61. Tarlov E, Schmidek H, Scott RM, Wepsic JG, Ojemann RG. Reflex hypotension following carotid endarterectomy: mechanism and management. J Neurosurg 1973; 39:323–327.
62. Mendelsohn FO, Weissman NJ, Lederman RJ, Crowley JJ, Gray JL, Phillips HR, Alberts MJ, McCann RL, Smith TP, Stack RS. Acute hemodynamic changes during carotid artery stenting. Am J Cardiol 1998; 82:1077–1081.

11

Opinions on Current Applications of Carotid Bifurcation Angioplasty and Stenting

Barry T. Katzen
Miami Cardiac and Vascular Institute, Miami, Florida

Considerable interest in carotid angioplasty and stenting has developed in recent years supported by excellent results from a variety of independent single-site investigators including Roubin, Henry and Amor, Wholey, and others. These results followed the pioneering work of Theron and Mathias in Europe as well as Tsai in the United States. The author's personal experience began in the late 1980s with rare use of transluminal angioplasty in patients with critical carotid lesions who had absolute contraindications to surgical correction. It is reasonable to ask why more rapid acceptance of endovascular approaches to carotid artery occlusive disease has not occurred, despite such promising results. The following discussion is a review of the current status of carotid angioplasty and stenting in a multidisciplinary setting with the highest levels of quality assurance for both surgery and intervention, where competitive modalities are evaluated for safety and efficacy by multidisciplinary teams.

At this time, the Miami Cardiac and Vascular Institute (MCVI) has taken a relatively conservative approach to carotid intervention. Carotid stenting is performed by interventional radiologists who had historically done diagnostic carotid and cerebral angiography for both intracranial pathologies and extracranial occlusive disease. Both vascular and neurointerventionists are involved in performing procedures and all patients are evaluated by independent neurologists prior to and following therapy. Vascular surgery has had a skeptical if not obstructionist attitude, predominantly based on the outstanding results of carotid endarterectomy consistently obtained at MCVI. Neurology has had a conservative bias as well, but has accepted intervention as a real alternative in specific cases. Despite this environment, experience has been growing, albeit slowly.

Indications for therapy at MCVI reflect this conservative approach the patient accrual rate is relatively slow as a result. These indications are:

Symptomatic: Angiographic stenosis greater than 60%, high surgical risk defined by the North American Symptomatic Carotid Endarterectomy Trial (NASCET), restenosis of CEA sites, previous radical neck surgery or radiation, high bifurcation, contralateral occlusion

Asymptomatic: Angiographic stenosis greater than 85%, and the same parameters as for symptomatic patients

For any technique to be introduced to the medical armamentarium, data supporting safety and efficacy should

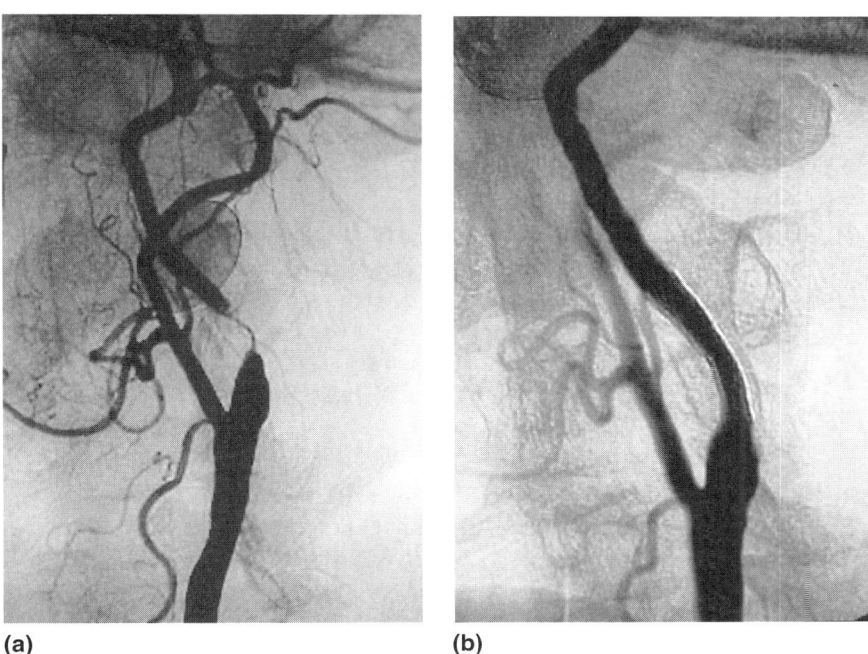

(a)   (b)

Figure 1 (a and b) An 84-year-old man with previous history of right-hemispheric stroke, with previous CEA, significant coronary artery disease, congestive heart failure, and who is found to have high-pitched bruit and "critical" lesion by colorflow duplex imaging. Stenosis measures 85% by NASCET measurement techniques. An 8 × 20 mm SmartStent was placed at 1 P.M. day 1, discharge was at 8 A.M. day 2, travel on vacation day 3.

be available, and in the case of carotid stenting, benefits should result in advantages over the status quo, i.e., standard surgical correction. At MCVI, 100% real-time quality assurance allows outcome analysis by impartial multidisciplinary panels, with unbiased medical records assessment by independent chart review. Surgical results for the past 3 years at the Institute have included stroke and mortality rate (combined) of less than 3%, creating an extraordinarily excellent target for a competitive therapy. In addition to excellent clinical outcomes, length of stay has averaged 1.1 days, and ICU usage occurs in less than 10% of patients. All of these results have resulted from physician directed "care mapping" and careful monitoring of outcomes.

Nonetheless, we believe carotid stenting (Fig. 1, a and b) will offer an important treatment alternative to carotid surgery, in particular when protection devices are available and proven to be effective. At that time, based on initial data, it is likely that the safety of carotid stenting may surpass that of carotid endarterectomy.

I. OPINIONS REGARDING CONSENSUS CONCLUSIONS

In general, the opinions expressed in the consensus panel results reflect the prevailing opinion of physicians at MCVI. I believe that there is a role for carotid stenting today in properly selected patients with clearly defined indications as indicated in the consensus summary. In low-risk patients, particularly those aged 55 or less, we are reluctant

---

Figure 2 (a, b, and c) A 70-year-old white man with previous history of CEA and amaurosis fugax associated with restenosis of the endarterectomy site. Although the carotid stenosis needs to be treated, careful assessment of the intracranial circulation shows probable old occlusion of the superior ophthalmic artery with abundant intracranial atherosclerosis.

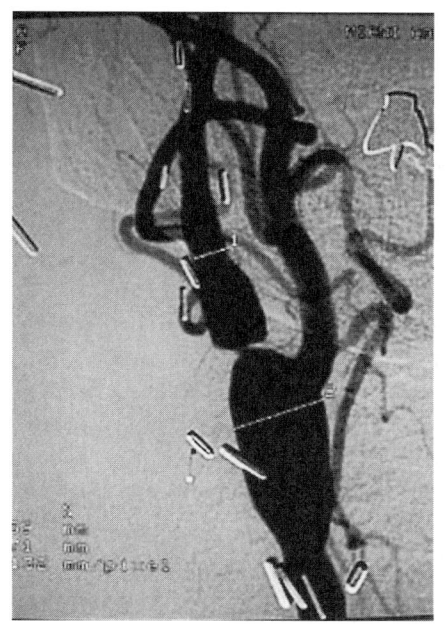 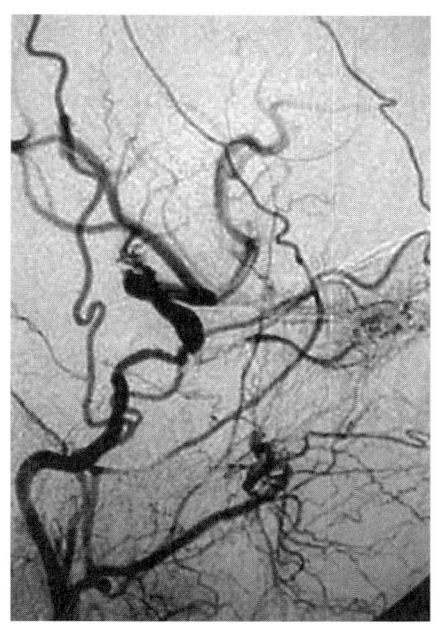

(a) **(b)**

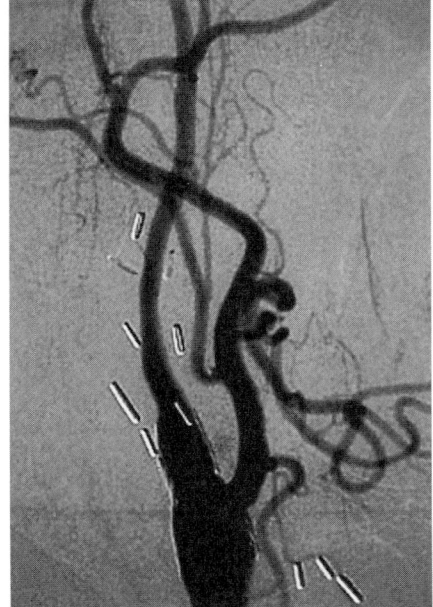

(c)

to use stenting as a treatment of choice. A perfect example is a patient who was recently referred for consideration for stenting for bilateral "critical" stenoses at a well-known and accredited noninvasive laboratory. He was evaluated by a surgeon who recommended CEA, and a second opinion was sought. The patient elected to proceed with possible stenting, despite a conservative presentation of the benefits, and aggressive presentation of the unknown factors for long term. Most importantly, I told the patient that it might be possible that no therapy was warranted at this time, and in fact the angiogram demonstrated bilateral stenoses of less than 60%, and no invasive therapy was performed. This type of clinical anecdote is frequent in our experience and draws concern to wide use of CEA without angiography, and in particular to the hazards of using duplex alone (Fig. 2, a, b, and c) as an indicator for therapy in upcoming clinical trials.

In general, I am in agreement with the consensus and prevailing opinions, but believe that when techniques are refined, and mechanisms for cerebral protection are proven, there will be a safety and efficacy advantage to carotid stenting, which will ultimately become the procedure of choice. It will not totally replace CEA, just as other noninvasive procedures have not totally replaced standard surgery, because of anatomical and technical limitations in many patients.

12

The Efficacy of Various Protection Devices During Carotid Artery Stenting

The Key to the Maturation of Stenting

Takao Ohki and Frank J. Veith
*Montefiore Medical Center–Albert Einstein College of Medicine,
New York, New York*

I. INTRODUCTION

Balloon angioplasty with or without stenting (BAS) for the treatment of carotid stenosis has been investigated for the past two decades. However, this procedure has not received wide acceptance primarily because of the availability of excellent surgical therapy and the risk of embolic stroke (1,2). The perioperative stroke/death rate following carotid BAS ranges from 5.3% to 8.2% (3–7). These initial trial results have been criticized because of the high neurological complication rate (8,9).

The main cause of these perioperative neurological deficits is thought to be embolic particles released from the carotid plaque during BAS (10–12). As early as 1990, Theron, the pioneer of cerebral protection, developed and first advocated the use of a balloon protection device (12). The risk of embolization and the need for cerebral protection during carotid BAS was further confirmed by our studies, which analyzed the production of embolic particles during BAS performed in an ex vivo model utilizing human carotid plaques. The plaques were collected from patients undergoing standard carotid endarterectomy procedures (13,14). These studies demonstrated that echolucent plaques tended to generate more embolic particles than echogenic plaques. In addition, those lesions with higher degrees of stenosis were at higher risk for embolization. More importantly, embolic particles were consistently produced from all the plaques that were stented.

Since Roubin and colleagues have suggested that the long-term patency and stroke prevention rates for carotid BAS are good if perioperative stroke can be prevented (15), it is believed that this procedure will gain popularity by virtue of its minimally invasive nature. The present chapter describes the authors' views on carotid stenting, including the unique nature of the carotid bifurcation plaque, which can be either advantageous or disadvantageous for stenting. In addition, it also describes several methods to prevent distal embolization, which may be of paramount importance in performing successful carotid stenting.

A. Unique Features of the Carotid Bifurcation Lesion That Make It Favorable for Stenting

Certain target site characteristics determine whether interventional procedures such as percutaneous transluminal angioplasty (PTA) or stenting perform well or not. Based on the vast experience with these procedures performed in various parts of the body, one can identify four characteristics that predict good outcomes (16–19). These include the following.

The Size of the Vessel

It has been unequivocally shown that the size of the vessel one is treating affects outcome. PTA of large vessels such as the aorta has been shown to be extremely durable. Stenting of the common iliac artery is more durable than stenting of the external iliac or femoral arteries. This is also true in the coronary circulation.

The Length of the Disease

Short, focal disease does better in terms of patency than long, diffuse lesions, and this is true in both the coronary and the peripheral circulation. One reason interventional procedures do poorly in superficial femoral artery lesions is that they are seldom short and focal.

Occlusion Versus Stenosis

In general, success and patency rates are higher when one is treating stenotic lesions as opposed to complete occlusions. In addition, the complication rates are lower for stenotic lesions. Carotid bifurcation lesions are always stenotic.

High Flow Versus Low Flow

The amount of outflow distal to a given lesion also dictates the long-term durability. Lesions in arterial beds with low flow (high resistance) are more prone to subacute occlusion. The internal carotid artery is a high-flow vessel, which is another favorable factor for stenting.

B. The Unique Nature of the Carotid Bifurcation Plaque That Makes It Unfavorable for Stenting

The Carotid Bulb

The carotid bifurcation consists of a bulb that is unique and is not found elsewhere in the body. It is thought that this bulb plays a certain role in the pathogenesis of the carotid plaque (20). The bulk is also responsible for the large plaque burden compared with other lesions such as in the coronary, renal, and iliac arteries, where the plaque burden is much less. This plaque burden relates to the complex nature of the carotid plaque, such as extensive plaque hemorrhage, necrosis, and fibrosis (Fig. 1) (21). Both the large plaque burden and its complex nature are predisposed to giving rise to embolization following balloon dilatation and stent placement.

The Unique End-Organ

The end-organ that the carotid artery supplies blood to is probably the most sensitive organ to embolization. A small embolus, too small to be recognized on arteriography, can cause a severe neurological deficit. This is not the case with other lesions that are usually subjected to stenting.

Because of the two reasons cited above and because distal embolization is often irreversible, carotid stenting was not considered as a first-line treatment option despite the favorable factors mentioned earlier. However, if there is a way to prevent this important shortcoming, a carotid

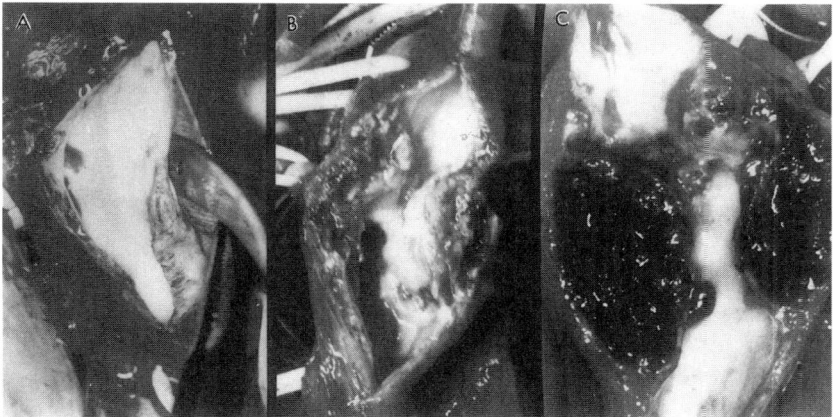

Figure 1 Macroscopic photographs of various carotid plaques. Carotid plaques may be fibrous (A), necrotic (B), or hemorrhagic (C). (From Ref. 21.)

bifurcation stenosis may be one of the most ideal lesions for balloon angioplasty and stenting.

II. BRAIN PROTECTION

There are three different approaches to brain protection (Table 1). We have had the opportunity to evaluate several distal protection devices using either the ex vivo human carotid stenting model (13,14) or canine models. This chapter describes the basic mechanism of various protection devices.

A. The PercuSurge GuardWire (PercuSurge, Inc., Sunnyvale, CA)

The GuardWire Temporary Occlusion Catheter (Fig. 2) (22) has an external diameter that is similar to commonly used 0.014-in. guidewires. Its shaft is hollow and it has a flexible,

Table 1   Various Approaches to
Brain Protection

1. Distal occlusion
      Theron balloon
      PercuSurge Guardwire
      Henry-Amor balloon
2. Distal filter
      MedNova NeuroShield
      EPI filter wire
      Angioguard filter
      SciMed Sentinel
      ArteriA Bate floating filter
3. Proximal occlusion
      Kachel balloon
      ArteriA Parodi catheter

shapable guidewire distal tip. An elastomeric occlusion balloon is located at the proximal end of the distal tip. The
GuardWire (with its deflated balloon) crosses the lesion
with minimal resistance (Fig. 3). Once the lesion is crossed,
an inflation device is attached to the proximal end of the
GuardWire catheter and the occlusion balloon is inflated
with dilute contrast agent. Following inflation of the occlusion balloon, an angiogram is taken to ensure complete occlusion (protection) of the distal carotid artery and to make
certain that no embolic materials can flow upstream (Fig.
3). The inflation device is then removed from the proximal
end of the wire while the occlusion balloon remains inflated,
thus providing coaxial exchange capability to the Guard-
Wire for PTA balloon and stent delivery catheters. With the
occlusion balloon inflated, balloon angioplasty and stenting can be performed to treat a stenosis in the internal carotid artery. Multiple embolic materials that are released
during BAS remain in the carotid bulb because of the
GuardWire occlusion balloon. Following removal of the angioplasty balloon catheter, an aspiration catheter (Export

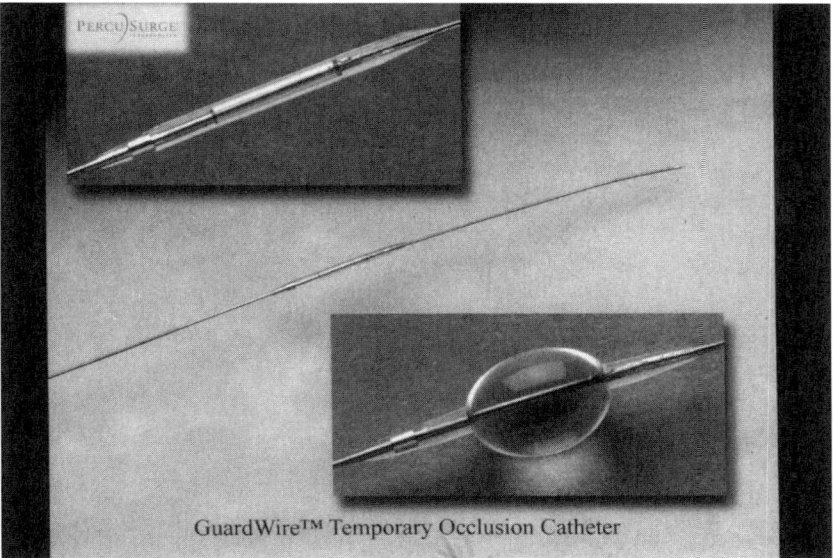

GuardWire™ Temporary Occlusion Catheter

Figure 2 The GuardWire Temporary Occlusion Catheter. The external diameter of the GuardWire is 0.014 in., which is compatible with preexisting catheters and balloons. It has a flexible, shapable distal tip. An elastomeric occlusion balloon is located at the proximal end of this tip. When deflated, the occlusion balloon has a diameter of 0.035 in., permitting smooth passage through even tight stenoses. Note the smooth, tapered transition zones at both ends of the elastomeric balloon.

PercuSurge, Inc., Sunnyvale, CA) is introduced over the GuardWire for aspiration of the embolic material. Loose embolic material that is trapped by the GuardWire occlusion balloon can be aspirated through the large lumen of the Export catheter (Fig. 4).

Initial experience with the GuardWire for the treatment of degenerated saphenous vein grafts in the coronary circulation has been very promising, and Food and Drug Administration approval for this application is imminent (23). Results of a feasibility study performed in Europe for the

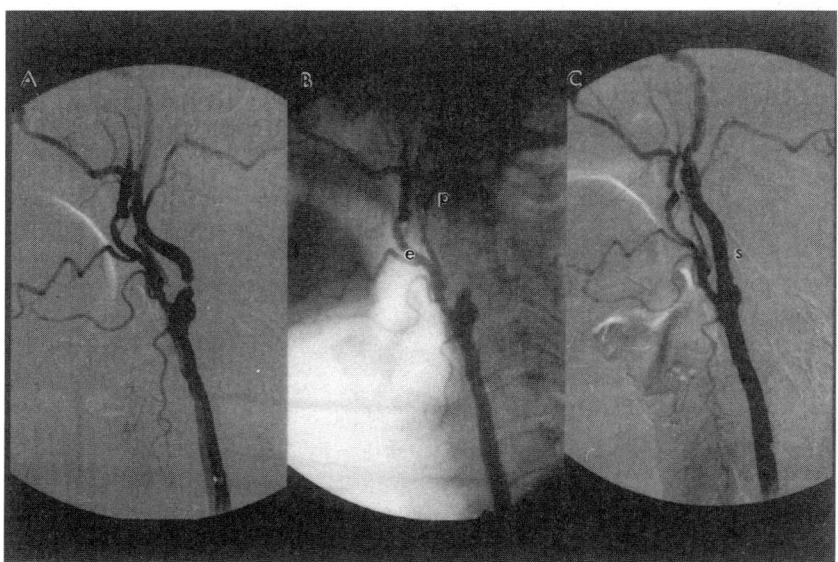

Figure 3 Angiograms of a patient with symptomatic carotid stenosis treated at Montefiore Medical Center. CEA was considered a prohibitive risk due to a history of multiple radiation treatments for a salivary gland tumor. (A) Preinterventional angiogram. Note the focal nature of the carotid plaque with normal, large-caliber distal and proximal arteries. (B) The GuardWire brain protection balloon (PercuSurge, Sunnyvale, CA) was used to prevent procedural embolic stroke. Once the occlusion balloon was inflated in the internal carotid artery distal to the lesion, complete occlusion of flow in the internal carotid artery was achieved. P: PercuSurge brain protection balloon (GuardWire); e: external carotid artery. (C) BAS was performed with a Wallstent (s) (Schneider, Minneapolis, MN) under brain protection. Completion angiogram shows good result. Multiple embolic particles were recovered with an aspiration catheter prior to deflating the GuardWire balloon.

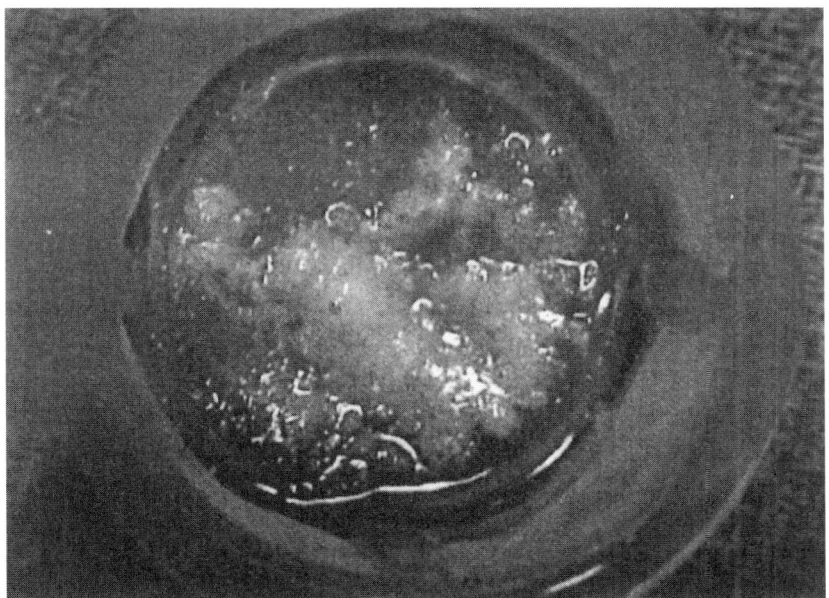

Figure 4 Macroscopic photograph of embolic particles that were recovered with the Export catheter. These embolic particles would otherwise have embolized to the brain.

carotid application have also been promising (24). This on-going study showed that there was only one minor stroke among 93 patients treated with carotid stenting under GuardWire protection. Only one patient could not tolerate balloon occlusion, and significant embolic debris was recovered in all cases (Table 2). Clinical trials in the United States were initiated in September 1999 at five centers including Montefiore Medical Center.

B. The MedNova NeuroShield (MedNova, Inc., Ireland)

The MedNova NeuroShield device is a temporary percutaneous transluminal intra-arterial filtration system. It is de-

Table 2 The Safety and Efficacy of the PercuSurge
GuardWire in the Treatment of Carotid Stenosis:
European Multicenter Trial (22)

Number of patients	93
Percent of neurological complications	
TIA	0
Minor stroke	1
Major stroke	0
Technical success, %	99[a]
Mean number of emboli recovered	76
Mean occlusion time	480 sec

[a] One patient did not tolerate balloon occlusion.

signed to conform to the vessel lumen and to capture emboli produced during BAS while maintaining flow (Fig. 5).
(25) The filtration element is mounted 2 cm proximal to the
distal tip of the 0.014-in. guidewire and it has large entry
ports at the proximal end and multiple perfusion pores at
the distal end. The filtration element contains a preshaped
nitinol expansion system that assists in filter deployment
as well as in fluoroscopic visualization. The system consists
of a delivery catheter, a filter guidewire, and a retrieval
catheter. The filter guidewire, which is encapsulated in the
delivery catheter, was introduced through the main port of
the sheath that was connected to the proximal end of the
carotid plaque in our ex vivo system. This filter guidewire
was passed through the stenosed carotid plaque after
which the delivery catheter was retracted, thereby deploying the filter in the distal internal carotid artery (Fig. 6). The
delivery catheter was then completely withdrawn and dis-
carded. Maintenance of flow through the filter was confirmed by injecting contrast (Fig. 6). An angioplasty balloon
was then inserted over this filter guidewire to the target lesion. Following predilatation, a stent was deployed across
the lesion. After completion of the procedure, the filter
guidewire was recovered using a retrieval catheter. The filtration element along with any captured embolic particles

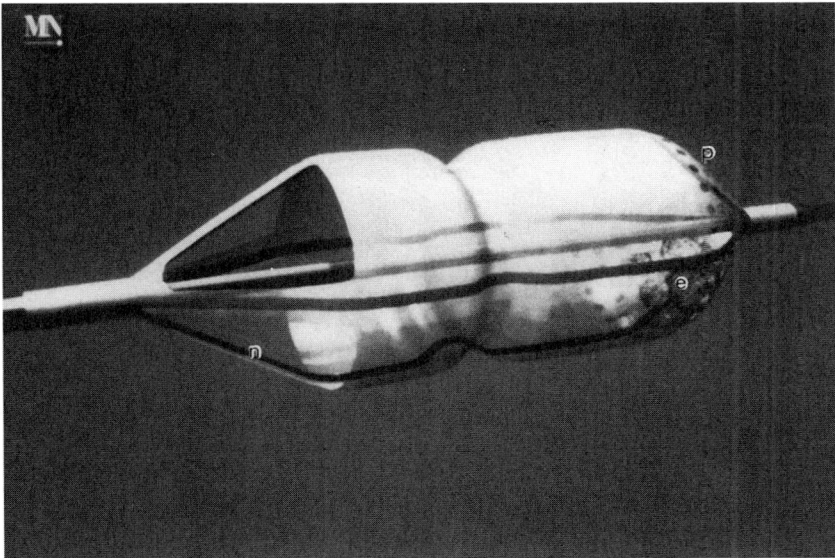

Figure 5   The MedNova NeuroShield. The filtration element has large entry ports at the proximal end and multiple perfusion pores (p) at the distal end. The filtration element contains a preshaped nitinol expansion system that assists in filter deployment as well as in fluoroscopic visualization. Abbreviations: e, emboli; n, nitinol.

was completely enveloped by introducing the large-bore retrieval catheter over the wire, and the entire device and its contents were then removed (Figs. 6,7). Initial clinical experience in four patients with carotid stenosis suggested the safety and efficacy of the NeuroShield filter (G. S. Roubin, personal communication). Clinical trials to evaluate the efficacy of this filter in the treatment of coronary and carotid lesions will be initiated in the United States before the end of the year 2000.

C.   The ArteriA Anti-embolization Catheter (ArteriA, CA)

The ArteriA balloon catheter is a guiding catheter with an occlusion balloon attached at the distal end of the catheter

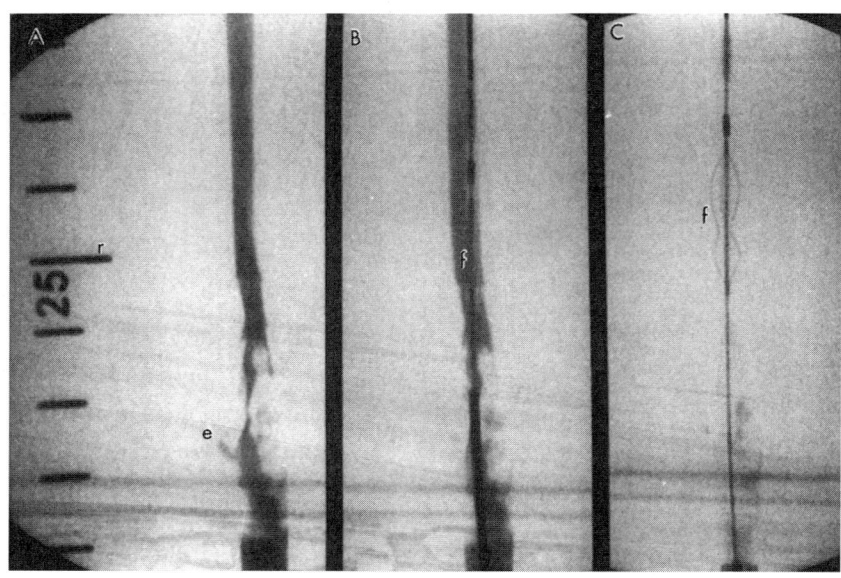

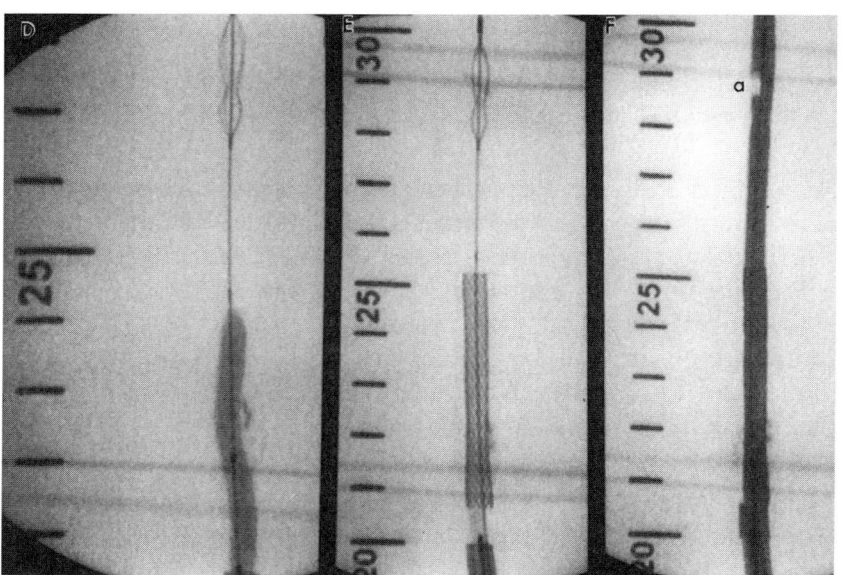

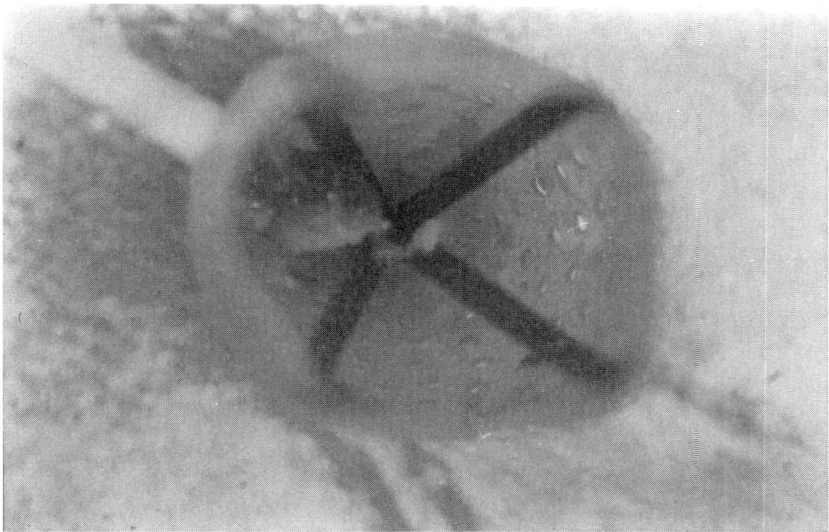

Figure 7 Close-up view of the inside of the filter following carotid artery stenting. Multiple embolic particles have been captured. (From Ref. 25.)

Figure 6 (A) Preinterventional ex vivo angiogram. A high-grade stenosis is seen in the internal carotid artery. The external carotid artery (e) is ligated. (r: radiopaque ruler.) (B) Initial filter guidewire passage through the stenosis was accomplished without difficulty because of the low profile and smooth transition between the tip wire and the delivery catheter. (f: nitinol-supported filter encased in the delivery catheter prior to deployment.) (C) Fluoroscopic image following filter guidewire deployment. Nitinol-supported filter (f) is fully deployed in the distal internal carotid. (D) Predilatation of the lesion is performed with a coronary balloon under filter protection. (E) A Wallstent is also deployed under filter protection. (F) Completion angiogram shows successful recanalization of the internal carotid artery. Flow through the filter is preserved. (a: embolus captured in the filter.) (From Ref. 25.)

(Fig. 8) (26). It is equipped with a dilator that allows safe and smooth insertion into the common carotid artery over a wire. This catheter has two lumens, one of which is for the insertion of an external carotid occlusion balloon. The main lumen has an inner diameter of 7 Fr, which allows the passage of balloons and stents. Once the ArteriA catheter is inserted into the common carotid artery, the occlusion balloon, which is located on the outer surface of the catheter, is inflated, thereby occluding inflow to the carotid bifurcation while maintaining access to the carotid bifurcation lesion through the main lumen. The side port of the ArteriA catheter can then be connected to a sheath that is percutaneously inserted into the femoral vein. This creates a temporary artery-to-vein shunt, which causes reversal of flow in the common carotid artery and its branches (Fig. 9). Any particles that are released will flow through the ArteriA catheter and will be captured by a filter that is placed between the artery-vein connection. In cases in which this re-

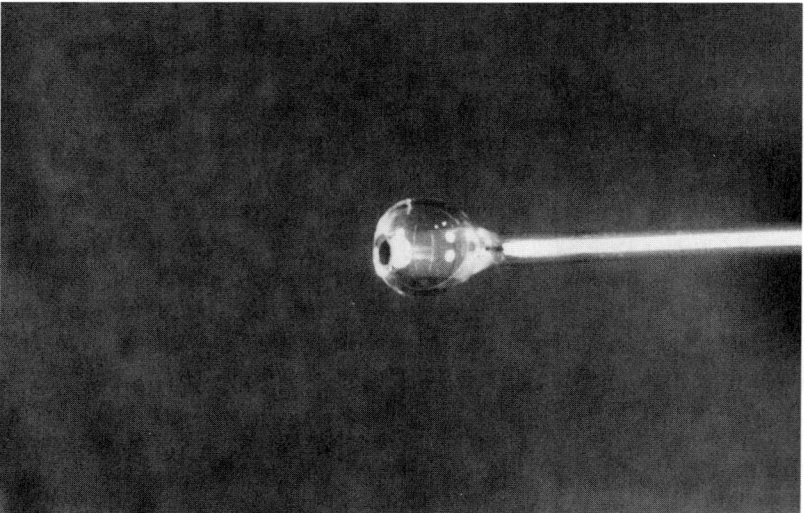

Figure 8 Close-up view of the ArteriA Parodi antiembolization catheter.

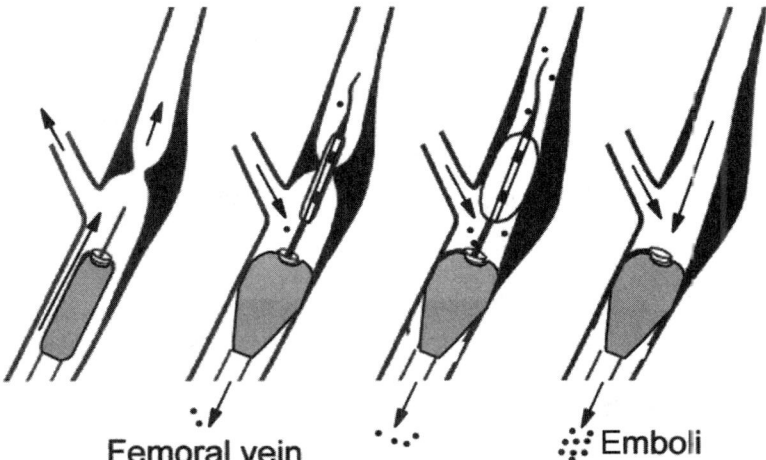

Femoral vein   Emboli

Figure 9 Mechanism of the ArteriA proximal occlusion balloon catheter used for the prevention of emboli. The reversal of flow can be achieved prior to manipulating the fragile carotid plaque. An alternative method is to occlude the external carotid artery with the specially designed low-profile occlusion balloon.

versal of flow cannot be achieved, a low-profile external artery occlusion balloon is inserted through the second lumen of the catheter into the external carotid artery. This step is required to prevent retrograde flow through the external carotid artery that potentially might cause prograde internal carotid artery flow, which could carry emboli to the brain. Once either of these techniques is employed, one can safely perform BAS. Ten carotid stenoses were treated under ArteriA catheter protection in Argentina, and technical success was achieved in all cases. No neurological events occurred in these 10 patients (J. C. Parodi, personal communication).

D. EPI Filter Wire (Embolic Protection Inc., San Carlos, CA)

The EPI filter wire is unique in that it has an off-center filter attached to a guidewire. Because of the unique design of

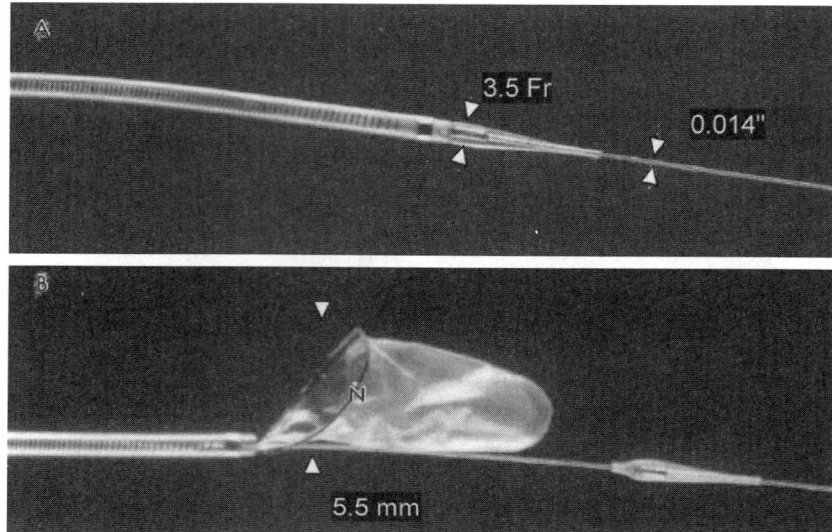

Figure 10 (A) EPI filter wire. Note the low profile (3.5 Fr) and the smooth transition tip of the EPI filter wire. (B) Deployment mechanism of the EPI filter wire. Once the outer sheath is retracted, the off-center, oval-shape nitinol frame (N) opens and assures complete contact of the filter against the arterial wall.

the "fish-mouth" filter opening, it is extremely flexible and also has a low crossing profile (3.5 Fr) (Fig. 10). In addition, the nitinol framework that supports the filter provides complete circumferential contact with the arterial wall, thereby assuring complete apposition of the filter, even in diseased and tortuous vessels. Finally, this filter can be recaptured (collapsed) and retrieved using any standard peripheral balloon that is used for the post dilatation. This will certainly simplify the procedure as opposed to using a special retrieval catheter.

E.   Other Devices

Other devices are being developed, including the Angio-Guard filter (AngioGuard, Inc., Cordis, Warren, NJ) and the

Sentinel filter (Boston Scientific Corporation, SciMed, Minneapolis, MN).

III. COMMENTS

One of the major drawbacks of carotid BAS is the relatively high incidence of periprocedural neurological events. Otherwise, the midterm results appear to be promising, and the minimally invasive nature of this technique is apparent (15). Therefore, if perioperative neurological events can be prevented with the use of these distal protection devices, carotid bifurcation stenosis may be one of the most ideal lesions for balloon angioplasty and stenting.

Another issue related to carotid BAS is the lack of a dedicated, optimal stent. All studies reported in the literature have used either a Palmaz stent or a Wallstent, both of which were not designed or approved for this particular procedure (3–7,15). However, several companies are currently involved in designing a stent specifically for carotid use, and some of these stents are undergoing phase 1 or 2 clinical trials. It will not be long before a dedicated, more ideal stent will be available.

Carotid endarterectomy is the most commonly performed major vascular operation in the United States— 150,000 cases are performed in the United States annually and 300,000 are performed worldwide. This signature operation for vascular surgeons may indeed be replaced with BAS once the aforementioned issues are settled. A brain protection device may play a key role in the transition of how patients with carotid stenosis are treated. At this time, it is not clear which system will perform best, but based on our experimental studies and the initial clinical experiences, they all appear to be promising. For those who are currently not performing carotid BAS, it may be ethical and reasonable to wait until these promising devices become available. For those who are performing carotid BAS, it would seem reasonable to aggressively move to some form of brain protection.

ACKNOWLEDGMENTS

This study was supported by grants from the James Hilton Manning and Emma Austin Manning Foundation, the Anna S. Brown Trust, and the New York Institute for Vascular Studies.

REFERENCES

1. North American Symptomatic Carotid Endarterectomy Trial Collaborators. Beneficial effect of carotid endarterectomy in symptomatic patients with high-grade carotid stenosis. N Engl J Med 1991; 325:445–453.
2. Executive Committee for the Asymptomatic Carotid Atherosclerosis Study. Endarterectomy for asymptomatic carotid artery stenosis. JAMA 1995; 273:1421–1428.
3. Iyer SS, Roubin GS, Yadav JS, et al. Extra-cranial carotid artery stenting: balloon expandable versus self expanding stents. Circulation 1996; 93(suppl. 1):1–383.
4. Diethrich EB, Ndiaye M, Reid DB. Stenting in the carotid artery: initial experience in 110 patients. J Endovasc Surg 1996; 3:42–62.
5. Henry M, Amor M, Henry I, et al. Endovascular treatment of atherosclerotic internal carotid artery stenosis. J Endovasc Surg 1997; 4(suppl 1):1–14.
6. Bergeron P, Chambran P, Hartung O, Bianca S. Cervical carotid artery stenosis: which technique, balloon angioplasty or surgery? J Cardiovasc Surg 1996; 37(suppl 1–5):73–75.
7. Wholey MH, Eles G, Jarmolowski CR, et al. Percutaneous transluminal angioplasty and stents in the treatment of extra-cranial circulation. J Interven Cardiol 1996; 9:225–231.
8. McGuinness CL, Burnand KG. Percutaneous transluminal angioplasty of the internal carotid artery. Br J Surg 1996; 83:1171–1173.

9. Stanley JC, Abbott WM, Towne JB, et al. Statement regarding carotid angioplasty and stenting. J Vasc Surg 1996; 24: 900.
10. DeMonte F, Peerless SJ, Rankin RN. Carotid transluminal angioplasty with evidence of distal embolization. J Neurosurg 1989; 70:138–141.
11. Theron JG, Payelle GG, Coskun O, et al. Carotid artery stenosis: treatment with protected balloon angioplasty and stent placement. Radiology 1996; 201:627–636.
12. Theron J, Courtheoux P, Alachkar F, Bouvard G, Maiza D. New triple coaxial catheter system for carotid angioplasty with cerebral protection. Am J Neuroradiol 1990; 11:869–874.
13. Ohki T, Marin ML, Lyon RT, et al. Human ex vivo carotid artery bifurcation stenting: correlation of lesion characteristics with embolic potentials. J Vasc Surg 1998; 27:463–471.
14. Ohki T, Marin ML, Lyon RT, Veith FJ. An in vitro model for the assessment of carotid artery stenting. Endovasc Multimedia Rev 1997; 3:5–8.
15. Liu MW, Roubin GS, Mathur A. Neurological events after successful carotid stenting (abstr). JACC 1998; 31(suppl A): 64A.
16. Ahn SS, Rutherford RB, Becker GJ, et al. Reporting standards for lower extremity arterial endovascular procedures. Society for Vascular Surgery/International Society for Cardiovascular Surgery. J Vasc Surg 1993; 17:1103–1107.
17. Pentecost MJ, Criqui MH, Dorros G, et al. Guidelines for peripheral percutaneous transluminal angioplasty of the abdominal aorta and lower extremity vessels. A statement for health professionals from a special writing group of the Councils on Cardiovascular Radiology, Arteriosclerosis, Cardio-Thoracic and Vascular Surgery, Clinical Cardiology, and Epidemiology and Prevention, the American Heart Association. Circulation 1994; 89(1):511–531.
18. Johnston KW. Factors that influence the outcome of aortoiliac and femoropopliteal PTA. Surg Clin North Am 1992; 72: 843–850.
19. Laborde JC, Palmaz JC, Rivera FJ, et al. Influence of anatomic distribution of atherosclerosis on the outcome of re-

vascularization with iliac stent. Journal of Vascular Interventional Radiology 1995; 6:513–521.

20. Zarins CK, Giddens DP, Bharadvaj BK, et al. Carotid bifurcation atherosclerosis. Quantitative correlation of plaque localization with flow velocity profiles and wall shear stress. Circ Res 1983; 53(4):502–514.

21. Imparato AM. Carotid pathology. In: Veith FJ, Hobson RW II, Williams RA, Wilson SE, eds. Vascular Surgery. Principles and Practice. New York: McGraw-Hill, 1987:623–635.

22. Ohki T, Veith FJ. The potential of the Percusurge Guardwire to prevent embolic events in endovascular interventions. Endocardiovas Multimedia Mag 1998; 2:33–38.

23. Webb JG, Carere RG, Virmani R, et al. Retrieval and analysis of particulate debris after saphenous vein graft intervention. J Am Coll Cardiol 1999; 34(2):468–475.

24. Henry M, Amor M. The safety and efficacy of the PercuSurge GuardWire in the treatment of carotid stenosis: European multi center trial. Presented at the 11th Transcatheter Cardiovascular Therapeutics meeting, Washington, DC, October 22–25, 1999.

25. Ohki T, Roubin GS, Veith FJ, Iyer SS, Brady E. The efficacy of a filter device in preventing embolic events during carotid artery stenting: an ex-vivo analysis. J Vasc Surg 1999; 30: 1034–1044.

26. Ohki T, Parodi JC, Bates M, et al. The need for protection device during carotid artery stenting. Presented at the 11th Transcatheter Cardiovascular Therapeutics meeting, Washington, DC, October 22–25, 1999.

13

Carotid Stenting

Results and Current Perspectives from a High-Volume Center

Nadim Al-Mubarak, Gary S. Roubin, Sriram S. Iyer, Jiri J. Vitek, and Gishel New
Lenox Hill Heart and Vascular Institute of New York, New York, New York

I. INTRODUCTION

Carotid stenting continues to evolve as an endovascular alternative to carotid endarterectomy (CEA) for patients with carotid artery stenosis. The procedure has gained widespread acceptance since its introduction especially in the treatment of patients at high risk from endarterectomy. Favorable outcomes have been achieved by many centers with reported procedural results that are well within the recommended guidelines for CEA practice (1–6). Clinical results continue to improve as the technique undergoes refinement. Neuroprotection devices and more suitable equipment are expected to further enhance the outcomes (7). Current data suggest that the time is suitable for prospective randomized trials that compare carotid stenting to CEA. The success of this comparison will depend on the ability of multiple medical centers and operators to master a technique the outcome of which is intimately related to the training and experience. There exists a marked learning curve associated with the clinical and technical skills required (8). This chapter describes our current approach to patient selection and the procedural details required to practice safe and efficacious carotid stenting.

II. SURGICAL BACKGROUND

The clinical significance of a least-invasive treatment approach to carotid artery occlusive disease is best understood in the context of current standard therapy, CEA. Based on three landmark multicenter, randomized trials comparing CEA to medical therapy, CEA is currently the standard therapy for symptomatic and asymptomatic extracranial carotid artery stenoses (9–15). The appropriate clinical indication for CEA, however, requires careful analysis of the population studied in these trials and the results obtained.

The North American Symptomatic Carotid Endarterectomy Trial (NASCET) represents the largest and most rigorously collected data with neurological oversight and provides a unique insight into the outcome of CEA when performed in centers of excellence (9,12,16). In this study, CEA combined with best medical therapy was clearly superior to medical therapy alone in reducing the risk of stroke in a select population with symptomatic extracranial carotid stenoses ≥ 50%. This benefit was directly related to the severity of the stenosis and was greatest for patients with stenoses ≥ 90%. The cumulative risk of any ipsilateral stroke at 2 years was 26% in the medical group versus 9% in the CEA group (absolute risk reduction of 17%). The overall combined 30-day rate of stroke and death in the CEA group was 6.7%. This increased to 14% in patients with an occluded contralateral carotid artery.

The second important study that examined the benefit of CEA in symptomatic patients was the ECST (1). This large randomized, controlled study demonstrated a clear benefit of surgery over medical management. At 3 years, the risk of stroke and death in the control group was 26.5% compared to 14.9% in the CEA group. In a subgroup analysis, however, a significant benefit was observed only in the male population. The overall 30-day incidence of stroke and death in the surgical arm of the ECST was similar to that seen in NASCET, but was higher in women (10.6%), in patients with systolic blood pressure ≥ 180 mmHg (12.3%), and in the presence of peripheral vascular disease (12.3%).

The ACAS investigation also showed clear benefit of CEA plus medical therapy in patients with asymptomatic extracranial carotid stenoses ≥ 60% (10). The cumulative risk over 5 years for ipsilateral stroke or any periprocedural stroke or death was 5.1% for the CEA group versus 11% in the medical group, again with the benefit not being significant in women. In this study, the estimated 30-day perioperative risk of stroke or death was 2.7%. Similarly, the population in this study was at low risk for CEA as important common comorbid conditions were excluded.

In 7% of patients (NASCET, ESCT) the CEA procedure was complicated by cranial nerve palsies, and in 13% there were a variety of local wound problems or medical complications (congestive heart failure, myocardial infarction, and cardiac arrhythmias) (7,9,11,12). These operative complications are important since they are negligible in patients undergoing carotid stenting.

Despite the benefit observed in these trials, the results cannot be extrapolated to the general population, largely because the risks of CEA are likely to be significantly higher in the populations excluded. These include patients with common conditions such as prior ipsilateral CEA, patients with significant coexisting coronary artery disease, as well as those with significant renal, hepatic, or pulmonary comorbidities. Numerous observational studies have reported increased rates of perioperative stroke and death in these groups (17–22). In addition, patients who underwent CEA in the presence of an occluded contralateral carotid artery had high perioperative combined stroke and death rates (14%) (9). Therefore, the perceived benefit of CEA in these patients may not be the same as that seen in the randomized population.

Furthermore, these trials were conducted by preselected high-volume surgeons who qualified for participation only if they demonstrated low perioperative stroke or death rates (9). Recent data, however, have shown definitive evidence that the actual incidence of stroke and death from CEA in the community is much higher than those reported in the randomized trials (15,23–25). Data from Medicare mortality statistics also showed that in-hospital mortality (not the more rigorous 30-day neurological assessment) was significantly higher in low-volume CEA centers than in the high-volume centers, and mortality in the latter was higher than in NASCET/ACAS centers (2.5%, 1.9%, and 1.4%, respectively) (25). Approximately 80% of CEAs in the United States are performed in low-volume hospitals by operators with less than 20 procedures annually (23). Moreover, published CEA outcomes are greatly influenced by the manner in which they are reported; specifically, strokes reported by single surgeons were lower (2.2%) than those reported when neurologists were involved in the authorship (7.7%) (26,27).

Accepting these limitations, the American Heart Association has set guidelines for the performance of CEA. According to these guidelines, CEA should be performed only if the combined stroke and death rates can be kept ≤6% in symptomatic and ≤3% in asymptomatic patients with severe extracranial carotid stenoses (28).

III. RATIONALE FOR ENDOVASCULAR THERAPY

The documentation of a significant incidence of both neurological and nonneurological complications associated with CEA in the landmark studies emphasizes the need to pursue an alternative safer method for treating carotid bifurcation disease especially in subsets of patients thought to be at higher risk from CEA.

Carotid artery stenting as an endovascular, less-invasive treatment approach offers several advantages. The majority of CEAs are still done under general anesthesia with recognized attendant risk especially from the frequently coexisting coronary artery disease or heart failure. Neurological complications are only apparent following recovery from anesthesia. In contrast, stenting is performed in a nonsedated conscious patient, where neurological changes are immediately recognized, and diagnostic intracranial angiography and appropriate therapeutic measures can be promptly initiated.

CEA is difficult in patients with high carotid stenoses or bifurcations, those with proximal/ostial common carotid lesions, and patients with short, obese necks, and requires extensive exposure of the carotid artery, adding considerable risk to the procedure. Patients with prior neck radiation for head and neck cancers and prior radical neck dissections also represent a challenge for the surgeon due to unusual locations of the lesions and extensive fibrosis in and around the arterial wall. Similarly, patients with restenosis after prior CEA are sometimes at higher risk for CEA due to scarring. These conditions usually require general anesthesia and some may require mobilization of the mandible. It is also more difficult for the surgeon to expose the artery for shunt placement. Fibrosis and scarring external to the artery require extensive dissection increasing the risk for cranial nerve injuries and prolonged wound healing. In some patients CEA cannot be performed and an interposition graft might be required. Generally, none of the above conditions are a problem for the endovascular approach and accordingly, carotid stenting may clearly be preferable for these patients (2,29–31). In addition, there are the potential advantages of a shorter hospital stay, shorter recovery, and reduced costs with stenting.

IV. PATIENT SELECTION

The current indications for carotid stenting are predominantly determined by the operator's experience and results. In general, there should be no contraindication to proceed with stenting provided the procedure can be performed with a combined stroke and death rate of ≤6% in symptomatic, and ≤3% in asymptomatic patients (32). Similarly, based on the current knowledge of the surgical outcome of carotid disease, stenting should only be applied to lesions that are ≥50% stenosis in symptomatic and ≥60% in asymptomatic patients (using NASCET angiographic measurements) (9–11,32).

The risk/benefit ratio of the procedure for any individual patient should be established prior to intervention. Based on our learning-curve experience and current technology, several factors associated with increased or decreased risk of procedural events have been identified (Table 1). However, as experience and technology improve, particularly with the application of cerebral protection devices, these factors may need to be revised.

During the initial learning curve of the operator, cases associated with higher periprocedural risk should be avoided and patients with low procedural risk should be se-

Table 1 Risk Status Associated with Carotid Stenting

Patients at increased risk for neurological complications
Clinical
1. Advanced age (>80 years)
2. Prior major disabling stroke
3. Cerebral atrophy/dementia
4. Unstable neurological symptoms (recent TIA or stroke)
Anatomical
1. Severely tortuous, calcified, and atherosclerotic aortic arch/arch vessels
2. Severe tortuosity just distal to the bifurcation
3. Coexisting proximal common carotid artery lesions
4. Total occlusion or long subtotal occlusions—"string sign lesions"
5. Severe concentric calcification
6. Angiographic evidence of a large thrombus
Patients at lower risk for embolic events
Clinical
1. Age ≤ 80 years
2. Less severe stenosis
Anatomical
1. Straight, noncalcified, "smooth arch vessels"
2. Nontortuous bifurcation
3. Absence of common carotid artery disease (except at adjacent bifurcation)
4. Absence of thrombus
5. Absence of kinks, loops, bend points at lesion site
6. Short lesions
7. Prior CEA

---

lected. These patients, especially those below the age of 80 years, can be stented with a low rate of periprocedural events (Table 4). The higher-risk subsets require much greater experience to achieve similar results. Our current practice is to treat only high-risk patients, especially the elderly, with adjunctive neuroprotection.

Although, at the beginning of the learning experience, there is a tendency to accept patients thought to be at higher risk for CEA, this temptation should be avoided if the patient has one or more of the higher-risk descriptors listed in Table 1. A number of high-risk situations for CEA, however, may be at low risk for stenting and represent ideal indications such as restenosis after prior CEA, or stenoses (2,17,31) in those with prior neck radiation and/or radical neck dissections (29,33). Patients with discrete proximal or ostial common carotid lesions, discrete lesions in the distal internal carotid artery, or lesions involving high bifurcations are also considered ideal candidates for stenting.

It must be emphasized that unfavorable lesion characteristics may only be apparent following initial angiography. The operator should be prepared to abandon the procedure at this point and consider elective CEA or continuing medical management. Operator judgement is critical in achieving low complication rates. Since there are usually reasonable alternative therapies, it must also be emphasized that failure to complete the procedure is acceptable but an avoidable complication is not.

V.   PERIPROCEDURAL CARE

Prior to the procedure, baseline neurological status and National Institutes of Health Stroke Scale (NIHSS) are documented by a neurologist. The carotid stenting procedure, the availability of alternative surgical therapy as well as the risks and benefits of each are carefully explained to the patient and family. In particular, we explain to our patients

(<80 years) that major complications are rare and occur in approximately 1%. We are able to note that we have not had a procedural death in the last 3 years. We discuss the risk of minor stroke (range: 1–4%), which may include minor weakness of a limb, mild confusion, or dysphasia, and that should this occur, complete recovery within a few days is usually the rule. We carefully point out that although our medium-term (5 years) outcomes appear favorable, long-term data are not yet available. We also inform patients that they will receive no sedation or general anesthesia and that the only discomfort will be related to local anesthesia at the vascular access site. Patients are started on antiplatelet therapy: soluble aspirin 325 mg twice daily (with meals) and Clopidogrel 75 mg every day preferably for 5 days prior to the procedure. In all cases, patients should have received a *total* dose of 450 mg of Plavix at least 3 h prior to the intervention. Standard hematological and chemical profiles are performed as well as an electrocardiogram. All medications are administered the morning of the procedure including antiplatelet therapy. Patients should be well hydrated prior to the procedure to minimize baroreceptor-induced hypotension and the rare risk of contrast nephrotoxicity.

In preparation for the procedure, patients should have good intravenous access and their head is cradled in a commercially available foam head constraint. Dentures and eyeglasses are removed. Atropine (0.6–1 mg) should be administered in all cases prior to intervention. Metaraminol, nitroglycerin, and dopamine are available for control of any hemodynamic instability that occurs. Standard resuscitation equipment is also available.

Continuous monitoring of the heart rate, arterial blood pressure, pulse oximetry, and electrocardiogram is mandatory throughout the procedure. Significant bradyarrhythmias and/or transient hypotension are not uncommon, especially when the bulb of the internal carotid artery is stretched (34). These usually recover spontaneously after balloon deflation. Occasionally, additional atropine (0.6–1 mg) is required for treatment of bradycardia or asystole. Hypotension is managed aggressively with fluid boluses, meteraminol (100–200 µg by bolus injection), and, if necessary, a dopamine infusion. In addition, the neurological status of the patient is frequently checked. This is achieved using a "squeeze toy" that is placed in the contralateral hand to monitor upper-extremity motor functions after each step in the procedure or by asking the patient to speak or move the contralateral foot. Loss of consciousness rarely occurs with balloon inflation, especially in situations when the ipsilateral hemispheric blood supply is isolated or if the contralateral carotid artery is occluded. This resolves spontaneously after prompt balloon deflation.

Following the procedure, the patient is observed in an interventional care unit with noninvasive hemodynamic monitoring. Vascular access site and neurological status are periodically observed. The sheaths are removed the same day when the activated clotting time (ACT) declines to ≤150 sec. Patients usually spend one night in the hospital. In our most recent experience femoral puncture sites have been closed on the procedure table with a 6F percutaneous arteriotomy suture system (Closure, Perclose Inc., Menlo Park, CA). This allows patients to ambulate shortly after the procedure, and facilitates same-day discharge in selected patients. In addition, early ambulation helps counteract the occasionally observed hypotensive effect of stenting on the carotid baroreceptors. If desired, patients can return to work and full activities after 3 days.

VI. PROCEDURAL TECHNIQUE

A complete four-vessel carotid angiogram with intracranial views is obligatory prior to stenting. This can be performed during the same sitting. Our current technical approach to the procedure can best be discussed in terms of: (1) accessing the carotid artery, (2) sheath placement, (3) predilatation, (4) stent deployment, and (5) postdilatation. The equipment required for carotid stenting is listed in Table 2.

A. Carotid Artery Access

In the majority of patients a 5Fr double-curve Vitek-catheter (VTK, Cook Inc. Bloomington, IN) (Fig. 1) is adequate to access the carotid arteries. The proximal curve of this catheter is opened and the tip, when located in the aortic arch, is pointing upward. This facilitates advancement of the 0.038 Glide-Wire (Boston Scientific Inc., Watertown, MA) even into severely tortuous brachiocephalic arteries. In the anteroposterior fluoroscopic projection, the catheter is placed in the upper thoracic aorta retaining its double curve with the tip pointing up to the left of the patient. From this position, gentle slow advancement of the catheter, retaining the

Table 2 Equipment for Carotid Stenting

5Fr Vitek catheter/100 and 125 cm long (VTK Cook Inc., Bloomington, IN)
0.038″/190-cm angle-tip Glide wire (Meditech Inc., Boston, MA)
7F/8F 90-cm Sheath (Shuttle, Cook Inc., Bloomington, IN)
0.038″/260-cm extrastiff straight wire (Amplatz, Cook Inc., Bloomington, IN)
0.014″/190-cm soft coronary wire (Balance, Guidant Inc., Temecula, CA)
4 × 40 mm, 0.018″-compatible balloon (COBRA, SciMed Inc., Maple Grove, MN).
0.018″/260-cm extrasupport wire (Roadrunner, Cook Inc., Bloomington, IN), or 0.014″/260-cm extrasupport wire (Stablizer-plus)
Self-expanding stents (Wallstent, SciMed Inc.; SMART, Cordis Inc.; Memotherm, Bard Angiomed Inc.; ACCULINK, Guidant Inc.; EndoTex, EndoTex Inc.)
Low-profile peripheral balloon catheter, 5 × 20 mm (Savvy, Cordis Inc., Miami, FL)

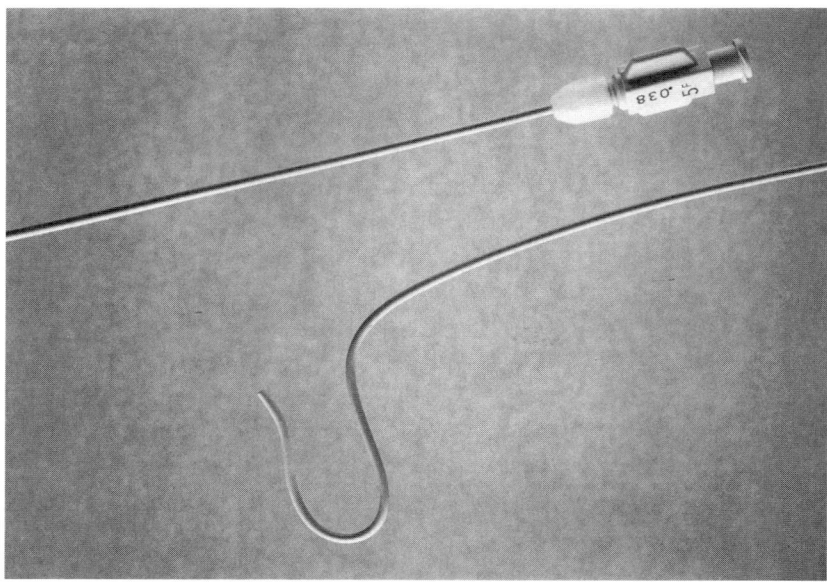

Figure 1 The 5Fr Vitek catheter facilitates catheterization of brachiocephalic arteries (VTK, Cook Inc., Bloomington, IN).

curved shape, engages it sequentially into the left subclavian, the left common carotid, and the innominate arteries. Slight rotation of the catheter within the innominate artery helps to distinguish between right common carotid and right subclavian arteries. If the catheter does not retain its shape, if it folds or twists to the right, the guidewire is used to reposition it.

After the origin of the target vessel is found, the Glide-Wire followed by the catheter is advanced into a stable position within the common carotid artery. To accurately direct the guidewire into the vessel, the catheter is gently rotated, pushed forward, or slightly retracted. If the wire starts to slip proximally, it is advanced cephalad. The wire should always enter the artery first, followed by the catheter, never the catheter alone. Advancing the catheter is performed by holding the wire while sliding the catheter slowly forward maintaining the wire distal inside the carotid artery. In very angulated origins, this maneuver is performed very slowly using push-pull/rotational maneuvers, taking advantage of the pulsating blood flow and the formation of a "favorable" supporting curve between the aortic arch and left upper thoracic aorta. A deep inspiration by the patient is often helpful. Medial rotation of the Glide-Wire tip while the catheter is in the innominate artery will direct it into the right common carotid. Road mapping is useful. In distended and elongated aortic arches, the origin of the left common carotid artery migrates posteriorly. In this situation, the catheter can be rotated so the tip of the catheter is located more posteriorly. In extremely dilated aortic arches, a sidewinder-curved (Simmons 3 curve) or HN5 catheters are occasionally required. It is essential to carefully backflush the catheter each time the Glide-Wire is removed and gently aspirate blood from the catheter to prevent air embolism. Small test injections are used to confirm the catheter position and exclude cather-induced dissections or flow impairment. A hand injection using a 6-ml control syringe with injection speed adjusted to the flow in the carotid artery is used (no more than 4 ml of 50% diluted contrast per injection).

B. Guiding Sheath Placement

If cerebral angiography has been performed in the same sitting, the target vessel is cannulated last and the 100-cm Vitek catheter is advanced over the Glide-Wire into the ipsilateral external carotid artery. Road mapping is useful. The Glide-Wire is then replaced with an extrastiff 0.038 exchange-length Amplatz wire (Cook Inc., Bloomington, IN). The Vitek catheter is then removed and a 7F/90-cm-long sheath (Shuttle, Cook Inc.) (Fig. 1B) is then advanced into the common carotid artery over the Amplatz wire and positioned just below the stenosis. The sheath (outer diameter: 3 mm/9F) is thin-walled, kink- and pressure-resistant with good flexibility and can accommodate 7F-outer-diameter devices. A similar 6F sheath is currently available for use with newer lower-profile devices. An open-ended Tuohy-Borst manually adjusting valve permits unimpeded catheter or guidewire introduction and the side arm allows flushing and contrast injection as well as continuous intra-arterial blood pressure monitoring (Fig. 2). The inner dilator facilitates its smooth introduction into the femoral and carotid artery.

If cerebral angiography has previously been performed and the target lesion is known, 6F close device sutures (Closure, Perclose Inc., Menlo Park, CA) are first deployed at the 5F puncture site. An exchange wire is introduced before removal of the close system and the guiding sheath is then positioned in the midthoracic aorta. A 125-cm Vitek catheter is introduced to access the carotid artery. Care must be

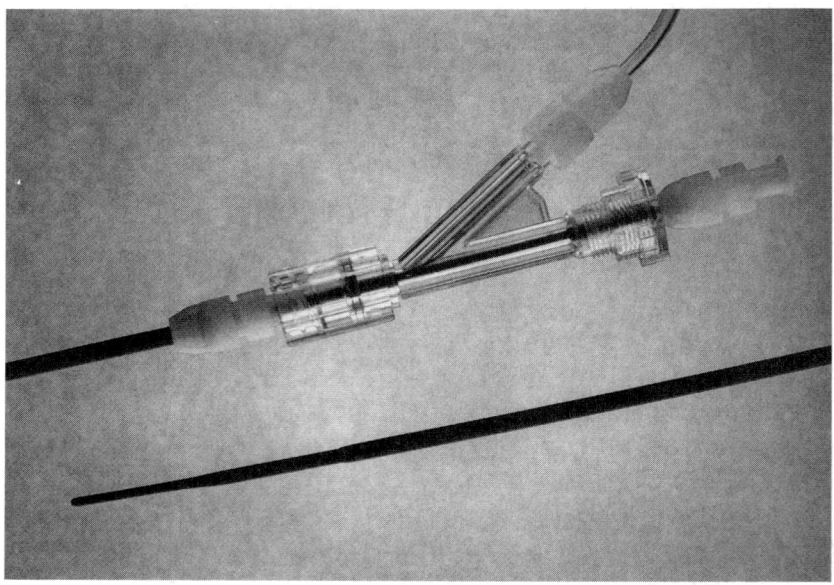

Figure 2   The guiding sheath used for carotid intervention (Shuttle, Cook Inc., Bloomington, IN).

taken not to advance the sheath too close to the aortic arch as this may decrease the maneuverability of the Vitek catheter. The target artery is then catheterized with the Vitak catheter and the sheath is placed as previously described. In the majority of cases the sheath can be advanced over the Vitek catheter–Glide-Wire combination without the need for an Amplatz wire. At this point, a heparin bolus (5000–6000 units) is given through the sheath. We do not routinely administer the IIb/IIIa platelet inhibitors for carotid stenting. A preinterventional angiogram is then performed at an angulation that best separates the internal and external carotid arteries and identifies bony landmarks, but not necessarily demonstrating the maximum stenosis severity. One should be aware that when the guiding sheath is placed in the common carotid artery, particularly if the carotid artery is tortuous, the vessel can be displaced upward and kinks can be formed in the internal carotid artery. These kinks disappear once the sheath is withdrawn.

C. Predilatation

The carotid stenosis is crossed with a steerable 0.018-in. coronary guidewire that is advanced to the base of the skull. For predilatation of the stenosis, we routinely use a 0.018-in. compatible, 4 mm × 40 mm coronary balloon (Cobra, SciMed Inc., Maple Grove, MN). If the stenosis is preocclusive, the lesion is first crossed with 0.014-in. soft coronary wire (Balance, ACS Inc., Santa Clara, CA) and then predilated with a 2.0 × 40 mm balloon (Ranger, SciMed Inc., Maple Grove, MN). A second dilatation, using the 4-mm balloon, is then performed. The Cobra-Balloon catheter is then advanced distally into the internal carotid artery and the 0.014-in. wire is changed for 0.018-in. exchange wire (Roadrunner, Cook Inc., Bloomington, IN) to facilitate stent positioning. In nontortuous internal carotid arteries, extrasupport 0.014-in. wire (e.g., Stabilizer-plus, SciMed

Inc., Maple Grove, MN) with a low-profile balloon (Ranger, SciMed Inc., Maple Grove, MN) can also be used as an alternative to an 0.018-in. wire system. Future 0.014-in.-compatible stents will be available (ACCULINK, Guidant Inc., Temacula, CA). More recently experience has been gained by crossing the lesion with 0.018-in. or 0.014-in. Percusurge balloon (Percusurge Inc., Sunnyvale, CA) or Neuro-Shield filter (MedNova Inc., Galway, Ireland) neuroprotection systems.

D. Stent Deployment

We have abandoned the use of balloon-expandable stents after the observation of stent deformities (35) with three exceptions: (1) stenting the ostium of the common carotid artery for more accurate stent placement, (2) treating the most distal segment of the internal carotid artery, and (3) when the self-expanding stent does not pass through a heavily calcified, "recoiling" lesion. Forcing the current high-profile delivery systems of the self-expanding stents embolizes plaque material. In this situation, a short balloon-expandable stent is first placed to prevent recoil before passage of a definitive self-expanding stent. If the stent does not pass through the stenosis, the lesion is predilated with a 5-mm balloon (Savvy, Cordis Inc.). The stent should never be forced across the stenosis. This problem will be solved using future lower-profile stent systems.

We now exclusively use self-expanding stents (Wallstent, Boston Scientific Inc.; SMART, Cordis Inc.; or Memotherm, BARD Inc.). These stents are easily deployed and, with few exceptions, only one stent is needed. The unconstrained diameter of the self-expanding stent to be deployed should be at least 1–2 mm larger then the largest vessel segment to be covered by the stent. We almost exclusively use one-size stents: for Wallstents (10 mm × 20 mm) and for the nonshortening Nitnol stents (10 mm × 40 mm). Oversizing the stent to the internal carotid artery has not been associated with late problems (36). Using vertebral bodies as landmarks, road-mapping, or contrast injections, the distal end of the stent is first placed within the healthy part of the internal carotid artery. The stent is then gradually released. It is not important where the proximal end of the stent will be located in the common carotid artery provided the stent has been adequately sized. Covering the external carotid artery with a stent does not cause problems. Recently, the nonshortening Nitinol self-expanding stents (ACCULINK, Guidant Inc., Temacula, CA; EndoTex, EndoTex Inc., Cupertino, CA) have been ideal for lesions that do not involve the carotid bifurcation. They can be precisely placed using the distal and proximal markers. An important technical point for the use of Nitinol stents is to release 3–5 mm of the stent distally and wait for the stent to expand fully and stabilize against the wall before further slow release of the rest of the stent.

E. Postdilatation

The self-expanding stent is postdilated with a 5.0 mm × 20 mm balloon. Using larger balloons increases the risk of carotid rupture and distal embolization. It is not necessary to produce a 0% residual diameter narrowing as residual stenosis of 10–15% does not cause hemodynamic problems. Importantly, it is not necessary to dilate the stent to obliterate segments of contrast-filled ulcerated areas external to the stent. This angiographic appearance is of no prognostic significance.

VII. CLINICAL RESULTS

Over the last 5 years, we challenged this new technique by treating a skewed, high-surgical-risk population that was excluded from prior randomized CEA trials (1,2,29–31,36–39). A large percentage of these patients were referred by physicians, including vascular surgeons, because of a variety of conditions that put them at higher risk for CEA (Table 3). These conditions include: prior ipsilateral CEA, prior ipsilateral neck radiation, contralateral occlusion, and severe coexisting coronary artery disease requiring staged/simultaneous carotid and coronary intervention. In addition, a variety of distal lesion locations, high bifurcations, and proximal common carotid artery disease were treated. All lesion subsets were attempted including severely ulcerated or calcified lesions, long severe lesions, "string sign lesions," and completely occluded vessels. Similarly, all types of severely diseased aortic arch vessels including tortuous, calcified, atherosclerotic, and stenotic common carotid arteries were accessed to complete the procedure. Representative cases of our series are shown in Figures 3–5. In general, our patients were an older group (mean age: 69 ± 10 years) of patients who suffered from a number of comorbidities including coronary artery disease, hypertension, and diabetes mellitus.

From September 1994 through March 2000 we completed stenting of 700 hemispheres in 619 consecutive patients (Table 3). The overall 30-day stroke and death rate was 6.4%. The 30-day mortality was 1.1%, major disabling stroke rate was 0.9%, and minor disabling stroke rate was 4.4%. The technique has gained wide acceptance at present because major adverse events have been uncommon and

Table 3 Total Experience (September 1994–April 3, 2000)

	Patients ($n = 619$)	Hemispheres ($n = 700$)
Age (mean ± SD)	69 ± 9 years	
Events		
Minor stroke	31 (5%)	31 (4.4%)
Major stroke	8 (1.3%)	8 (1.1%)
Fatal stroke	3 (0.5%)	3 (0.4%)
Nonneuro death	5 (0.8%)	5 (0.7%)

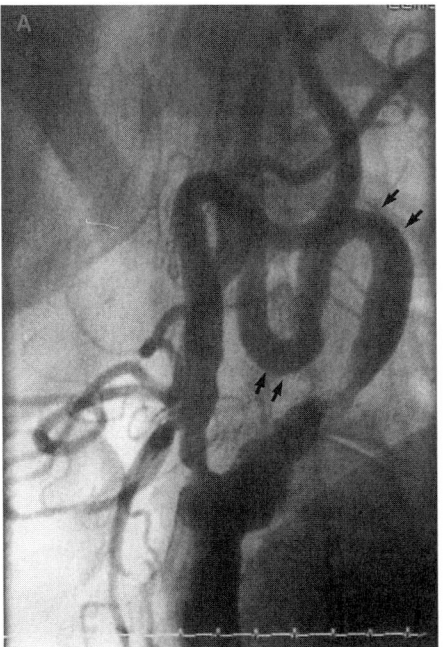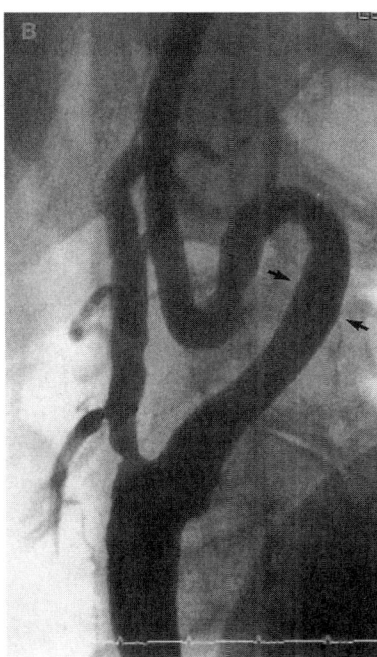

Figure 3 Case 1. Stenting of a tortuous carotid artery: (A) Preinterventional angiogram showing the lesion and the marked tortuosity of the internal carotid artery (arrows). (B) Poststenting angiogram. The distal end of the stent (SMART, Cordis Inc.) is placed just before the bend (arrow) without disturbing the anatomy. The stented site is widely patent.

minor strokes (usually only noted by detailed examination of the neurologist) have not been of functional significance to the patient.

Neurological events continue to be largely nondisabling strokes. Deaths and disabling strokes have been uncommon especially in patients <80 years. While embolic event rates in patients below the age of 80 years have been very low, patients ≥ 80 years have been associated with higher rates of neurological complications (Table 4). Preliminary results of neuroprotection devices appear to improve the outcome of stenting in this population.

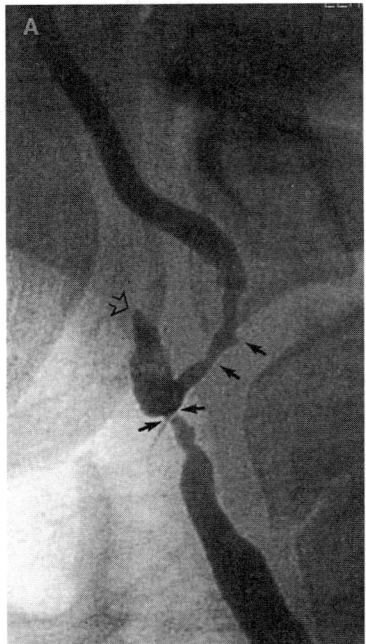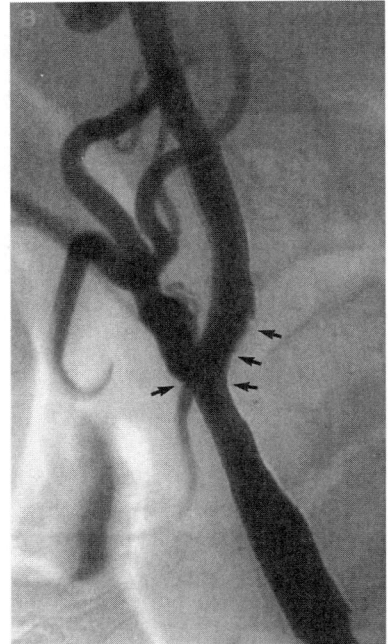

Figure 4   Case 2. Stenting of a severe lesion involving the carotid bifurcation and the proximal part of the internal carotid artery (thick arrows). (A) Preinterventional angiogram. The external carotid artery shows competitive flow (lined arrow) from collaterals via vertebral artery. (B) Poststenting angiogram: the carotid bifurcation is reconstructed (arrows) with good flow into the external carotid artery.

Figure 5   Case 3. Carotid stenting with neuroprotection. (A) Preinterventional angiogram showing severely narrowed origin of the internal carotid artery (arrow). (B) The occlusion balloon (arrows) (PercuSurge, PercuSurge Inc, Sunnyvale, CA). (C) Angiogram following deployment of a Wallstent (Boston Scientific Inc.). The origin of the external carotid artery is narrowed with good TIMI-III flow. This has not been shown to cause problems on follow-up.

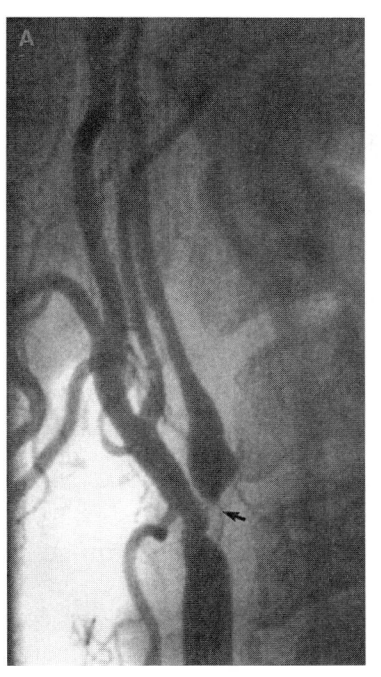

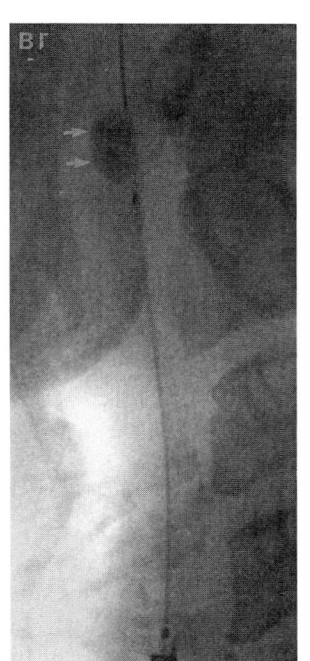

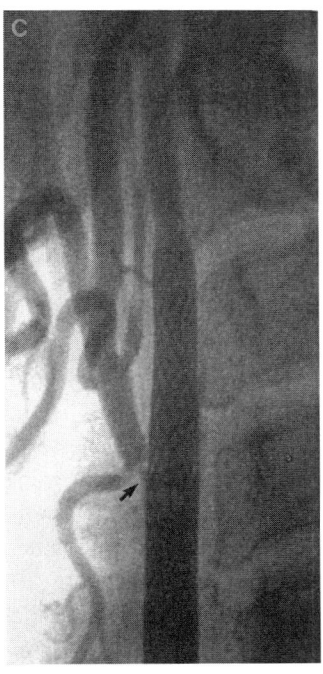

Table 4 Current Experience (November 1997–March 2000)

	<80 years	≥80 years	Total
Asymptomatic patients			
Patients/hemispheres	177/191	25/29	202/220
Minor stroke	2 (1%)	1 (3.4%)	3 (1.4%)
Major stroke	1 (0.5%)	2 (6.9%)	3 (1.4%)
Deaths	0	0	0
Symptomatic patients			
Patients/hemispheres	99/111	10/10	109/121
Minor stroke	4 (3.6%)	2 (20%)	6 (4.9%)
Major strokes	0	1 (10%)	1 (0.8%)
Death	0	0	0

Over the 5-year experience, we have modified our eligibility criteria. We now believe strongly that given current technology and taking into account the experience of the operator, careful patient selection is critical in maintaining low complication rates.

A. Current Experience

Current experience (November 1998 through March 2000) represents a consecutive series of elective carotid stent cases performed by this group at the Lenox Hill Heart and Vascular Institute of New York. The current results are shown in Table 4 and represent our experience in stenting with and without neuroprotection systems.

B. Learning Curve of Carotid Stenting

The results of carotid stenting are operator dependent and hence there exists a significant learning curve. Table 5 shows the periprocedural results of our annualized experience. The incidence of procedure-related major neurological complications has been low throughout the experience. The majority of these complications were isolated events directly related to practical technical decision making based

Table 5 Annual Progression of Experience (Periprocedural Events)

Years	9/94-9/95	9/95-9/96	9/96-9/97	9/97-9/98	9/98-9/99	9/99-3/00
Patients	86	96	118	83	145	76
Hemispheres	99	120	131	93	161	78
Minor strokes	7 (7.1%)	7 (5.8%)	7 (5.3%)	3[a] (3.2%)	5 (3.1%)	2 (2.6%)
Major strokes	1 (1%)	2 (1.7%)	1 (8%)	0	2 (1.2%)	1 (1.3%)
Fatal strokes	0	0	3 (2%)	0	0	0
Nonneuro deaths	1 (1.2%)	0	4 (3.9%)	0	0	0
All strokes/deaths	8 (8.2%)	10 (8.4%)	10 (7.3%)	2 (2.1%)	7 (4.3%)	3 (3.8%)

[a] One retinal artery embolus 2 weeks after the procedure.

on the nondedicated equipment availability and the operators' naïveté concerning patient selection factors. We have learned that these problems can be avoided by appropriate patient selection and careful technique. As a result, there has been a progressive fall in minor neurological events as the team experience has progressed.

C. Stent Restenosis

Of our first 225 successfully stented patients we were able to perform carotid follow-up angiography in 121 and follow-up duplex studies in an additional 29 patients. Of these 150 patients, restenosis (defined as 50% diameter narrowing) was present in eight (5.3%). Only four of these patients (2.7%) had restenosis that warranted repeat intervention. Restenosis in carotid stents can easily be treated with repeat balloon dilation. Similar rates for restenosis (6-month restenosis rate of 4.8%) were reported by Wholey et al. in a large multicenter registry. Furthermore, the late (>1 year) luminal loss following carotid stenting has been shown to be favorable (40).

D. Late Outcome

Systematic follow-up of our 528 patients (99.6%) with 604 successfully stented vessels at a mean of 17 ± 12 months (range 12–55 months) was obtained. There was an incremental 3.2% incidence of fatal and nonfatal stroke beyond 30 days. Freedom of fatal and nonfatal stroke at 3 years was $88 \pm 2\%$ and freedom of ipsilateral nonfatal stroke and all fatal stroke was $92 \pm 1\%$. The results compare very favorably with outcomes seen in the NASCET Trial.

VIII. FUTURE DIRECTIONS

It is now evident that many experienced operators can perform carotid stenting with low complication rates (3). Poor outcomes from carotid stenting, as with CEA, are related to technical skills and experience. In our view, the most successful results can be attained through collegial collaboration between cardiology, radiology, neuroradiology, and vascular surgery. There is an urgent need to train endovascular specialists who wish to perform this procedure. The next 5 years should be focused on education and technical training through symposia, workshops, and live demonstration courses. There is also an ongoing need to improve the equipment available for carotid stenting. Often, when we encounter a technical problem, it is attributed to the inadequacy of the devices currently available. There is a need for lower-profile stent delivery systems, better-access sheaths, and specially designed guidewires and balloons. It is likely that a variety of different stent designs will be required for optimal treatment of variable carotid bifurcation anatomy.

The major challenge from a technical perspective has been the development of "neuroprotective devices" that will reliably prevent any particulate matter that is produced during the intervention from embolization to the brain. Acherstaff and Jansen, using transcranial Doppler, showed that the number of embolic particles detected during CEA correlated with the rate of subsequent neurological events. Clinical experience (Theron) and work from the Ohki ex vivo model has shown that embolic particles can be released and captured during carotid stenting (41–43). The emboli can occur from aggressive guidewire manipulation, especially when using large-diameter guidewires, from balloon dilatation (particularly larger peripheral balloons), and during stent deployment and poststent dilatation (Ohki et al., unpublished results). Despite optimal treatment with antiplatelet therapy, embolic events occur invariably during the procedure, occasionally within 1–2 hr and very rarely within the 4 weeks following the procedure. Hence the application of cerebral protection during the procedure is expected to significantly decrease the risk of embolic events.

A number of neuroprotective devices are currently under evaluation in Europe and will be introduced to North
American centers in the near future. Two approaches are
under investigation, both of which provide distal protection
after careful passage of the lesion prior to definitive dilatation. One approach, first proposed by Vitek et al. (44) and
later pioneered by Jacques Theron (43,45,46), involves the
use of a distal occlusion balloon that interrupts flow during
critical maneuvers likely to release particles. The column of
blood containing embolic material is then aspirated using a
variety of techniques prior to deflating the balloon. Theron
reported an impressive reduction of embolic complications
from 8% to 2% using this technique. Theron's concept has
now been refined with more advanced technology, and a
number of distal occlusion, flush, and retrieval systems are
now under clinical investigation (Fig. 5) (7). This technique
might not be suitable for the 5–10% of patients with contralateral occlusion, critical contralateral disease, or an incomplete circle of Willis who may not tolerate prolonged carotid occlusion.

The second approach involves the deployment of an
atraumatic, low-profile embolic filter that is placed prior to
definitive lesion dilatation, and removed after completion of
stent positioning and expansion. The filter has the advantage of providing constant cerebral perfusion, allowing
more time for careful and precise intervention of the lesion.
Currently available devices are deployed and retrieved on
a 0.014-in. or 0.018-in. shaft that serves as the guidewire
for balloons and stent delivery system. They are user-
friendly and do not add significant time to the current procedure. Studies in ex vivo models using the NeuroShield
device (MedNova Inc., Galway, Ireland) have shown 90%
capture of particles of 200μ and 100% capture of particles
> 500μ (Ohki et al., unpublished results). Clinical trials are
currently in progress. Cerebral protection devices have the
potential to greatly enhance the safety of carotid stenting,
and when available, they will extend this specialized, less

invasive approach to the treatment of carotid stenoses to community-based interventionalists.

For carotid stenting to attain acceptance as a less traumatic, safe, and effective alternative to endarterectomy, it must be validated in a randomized controlled trial. One such trial, CAVATAS (47), has been completed; a second larger, NIH-sponsored study is planned, CREST (48).

CAVATAS, a prospective randomized controlled trial, was conducted in Great Britain through a collaborative effort between neurologists, radiologists, and vascular surgeons (47). In general, the trial included a high-risk, symptomatic population of patients with high-grade carotid stenosis. Inclusion criteria were much broader than in the NASCET trial and accordingly this study represents the first prospective evaluation of CEA in higher-risk patients with independent neurological assessment. The study was undertaken at large regional centers in Britain by experienced vascular surgeons. In contrast, the radiologists involved in the trial were operating within their learning curves for carotid intervention. Approximately 20% of the patients actually received stents (usually for "bailout" application). In addition, the stenting approach in this trial was suboptimal, inferior stents and large-profile peripheral balloons were used, and the technical approach with 0.035-in. wires without a guiding sheath was employed. Despite these differences in operator experience and the relative maturity of the techniques, both early and late outcomes were similar. The 30-day combined rates of major stroke and death were approximately 6% in both groups and 2-year neurological outcomes were identical.

CREST, a randomized controlled trial of CEA versus carotid stenting, plans to recruit 2500 patients with symptomatic stenosis $\geq$ 50% diameter narrowing (NASCET angiographic criteria). Primary end-points will be the incidence of death, any stroke and myocardial infarction at 30 days, and the incidence of ipsilateral stroke at 4 years. Rigorous credentialing of both surgeons and endovascular interventionists is currently ongoing to ensure that the trial is conducted according to the highest standards (49). Randomization is expected to begin in late 2000 when the credentialing phase is completed and participating interventionists demonstrate competency with carotid stenting procedure.

REFERENCES

1. Yadav JS, Roubin GS, Iyer S, Vitek J, King P, Jordan WD, Fisher WS. Elective stenting of the extracranial carotid arteries. Circulation 1997; 95:376–381.
2. Yadav JS, Roubin GS, King P, Iyer S, Vitek J. Angioplasty and stenting for restenosis after carotid endarterectomy. Initial experience. Stroke 1996; 27:2075–2079.
3. Wholey MH, Wholey M, Bergeron P, Diethrich EB, Henry M, Laborde JC, Mathias K, Myla S, Roubin GS, Shawl F, Theron JG, Yadav JS, Dorros G, Guimaraens J, Higashida R, Kumar V, Leon M, Lim M, Londero H, Mesa J, Ramee S, Rodriguez A, Rosenfield K, Teitelbaum G, Vozzi C. Current global status of carotid artery stent placement. Cathet Cardiovasc Diagn 1998; 44:1–6.
4. Shawl FA. Carotid stenting in patients with symptomatic coronary artery disease; a preferred approach. J Invasive Cardiol 1998; 10:432–442.
5. Diethrich EB, Ndiaye M, Reid DB. Stenting in the carotid artery: initial experience in 110 patients. J Endovasc Surg 1996; 3:42–62.
6. Mathias K. Stent placement in arteriosclerotic disease of the internal carotid artery. J Intervent Cardiol 1997; 10:469–477.
7. Henry M, Amor M, Henry I, Klonaris Ch, Chati Z, Masson I, et al. Carotid stenting with cerebral protection: first clinical experience using the PercuSurge guard wire system. J Endovasc Surg 1999; 6:321–331.
8. Iyer S, Roubin G, Vitek J, Bonomo R, Oetgen M, Lawrence E, Khanna A, Moussa I, Zucker D, Moses J, Yates V, Dean L. Four year experience with carotid stenting (abstr). J Am Coll Cardiol 1999; 33:21A.

9. North American Symptomatic Carotid Endarterectomy Trial. Methods, patient characteristics, and progress. Stroke 1991; 22:711–720.

10. Executive Committee for the Asymptomatic Carotid Atherosclerosis Study. Endarterectomy for asymptomatic carotid artery stenosis. JAMA 1995; 1421–1428.

11. European Carotid Surgery Trialists' Collaborative Group. MRC European Carotid Surgery Trial: interim results for symptomatic patients with severe (70–99%) or with mild (0–29%) carotid stenosis. Lancet 1991; 337:1235–1243.

12. North American Symptomatic Carotid Endarterectomy Trial Collaborators. Beneficial effect of carotid endarterectomy in symptomatic patients with high-grade carotid stenosis. N Engl J Med 1991; 325:445–453.

13. National Institute of Neurological Disorders and Stroke Stroke and Trauma Division. North American Symptomatic Carotid Endarterectomy Trial (NASCET) Investigators. Clinical alert: benefit of carotid endarterectomy for patients with high-grade stenosis of the internal carotid artery. Stroke 1991; 22:816–817.

14. Endarterectomy for moderate symptomatic carotid stenosis: interim results from the MRC European Carotid Surgery Trial. Lancet 1996; 347:1591–1593.

15. Mayo Asymptomatic Carotid Endarterectomy Study Group. Results of a randomized controlled trial of carotid endarterectomy for asymptomatic carotid stenosis. Mayo Clin Proc 1992; 67:513–518.

16. North American Symptomatic Carotid Endarterectomy Trial Collaborators. Barnett HJ, Taylor DW, Eliasziw M, Fox AJ, Ferguson GG, Haynes RB, Rankin RN, Clagett GP, Hachinski VC, Sackett DL, Thorpe KE, Meldrum HE. Benefit of carotid endarterectomy in patients with symptomatic moderate or severe stenosis. N Engl J Med 1998; 339:1415–1425.

17. Carotid angioplasty and stent: an alternative to carotid endarterectomy. Neurosurgery 1997; 40:344–345.

18. Akins CW. Combined carotid endarterectomy and coronary revascularization operation. Ann Thorac Surg 1998; 66:1483–1484.

19. Ballotta E, Da Giau G, Guerra M. Carotid endarterectomy and contralateral internal carotid artery occlusion: perioper-

ative risks and long-term stroke and survival rates. Surgery 1998; 123:234–240.

20. Bartlett FF, Rapp JH, Goldstone J, Ehrenfeld WK, Stoney RJ. Recurrent carotid stenosis: operative strategy and late results. J Vasc Surg 1987; 5:452–456.

21. Bass A, Krupski WC, Dilley RB, Bernstein EF. Combined carotid endarterectomy and coronary artery revascularization: a sobering review. Isr J Med Sci 1992; 28:27–32.

22. Borger MA, Fremes SE, Weisel RD, Cohen G, Rao V, Lindsay TF, Naylor CD. Coronary bypass and carotid endarterectomy: does a combined approach increase risk? A metaanalysis. Ann Thorac Surg 1999; 68:14–20.

23. Brott T, Thalinger K. The practice of carotid endarterectomy in a large metropolitan area. Stroke 1984; 15:950–955.

24. Cebul RD, Snow RJ, Pine R, Hertzer NR, Norris DG. Indications, outcomes, and provider volumes for carotid endarterectomy. JAMA 1998; 279:1282–1287.

25. Wennberg DE, Lucas FL, Birkmeyer JD, Bredenberg CE, Fisher ES. Variation in carotid endarterectomy mortality in the Medicare population: trial hospitals, volume, and patient characteristics. JAMA 1998; 279:1278–1281.

26. Rothwell PM, Robertson G. Meta-analyses of randomised controlled trials. Lancet 1997; 350:1181–1182.

27. Rothwell PM, Slattery J, Warlow CP. Clinical and angiographic predictors of stroke and death from carotid endarterectomy: systematic review. Br Med J 1997; 315:1571–1577.

28. Morey SS. AHA updates guidelines for carotid endarterectomy. Am Fam Physician 1998; 58:1898, 1903–1904.

29. Al-Mubarak N, Roubin GS, Iyer SS, Gomez CR, Liu MW, Vitek JJ. Carotid stenting for severe radiation-induced extacranial carotid artery occlusive disease. J Endovasc Ther 2000; 7:36–40.

30. Al-Mubarak N, Roubin GS, Liu MW, Dean LS, Gomez CR, Iyer SS, Vitek JJ. Early results of percutaneous intervention for severe coexisting carotid and coronary artery disease. Am J Cardiol 1999; 84:600–602.

31. Al-Mubarak N, Roubin GS, Vitek JJ, Gomez CR. Simultaneous bilateral carotid stenting for restenosis after endarterectomy. Cathet Cardiovasc Diagn 1998; 45:11–15.

32. American Heart Association. 1999 Heart and Stroke Statistical Update. Dallas, TX: American Heart Association, 1998.

33. Ahuja A, Blatt GL, Guterman LR, Hopkins LN. Angioplasty for symptomatic radiation-induced extracranial carotid artery stenosis: case report. Neurosurgery 1995; 36:399–403.

34. Al-Mubarak N, Liu MW, Dean LS, Gomez CR, Kretzer K, Alred D, Iyer SS, Vitek JJ, Roubin GS. Incidence and outcomes of prolonged hypotension following carotid artery stenting (abstr). J Am Coll Cardiol 1999; 33:65A.

35. Mathur A, Dorros G, Iyer SS, Vitek JJ, Yadav SS, Roubin GS. Palmaz stent compression in patients following carotid artery stenting. Cathet Cardiovasc Diagn 1997; 41:137–140.

36. Piamsomboon C, Roubin GS, Liu MW, Iyer SS, Mathur A, Dean LS, Gomez CR, Vitek JJ, Chattipakorn N, Yates G. Relationship between oversizing of self-expanding stents and late loss index in carotid stenting. Cathet Cardiovasc Diagn 1998; 45:139–143.

37. Roubin GS, Yadav S, Iyer SS, Vitek J. Carotid stent-supported angioplasty: a neurovascular intervention to prevent stroke. Am J Cardiol 1996; 78:8–12.

38. Al-Mubarak N, Roubin GS, Gomez CR, Liu MW, Terry J, Lyer SS, Vitek JJ. Carotid artery stenting in patients with high neurologic risks. Am J Cardiol 1999; 83:1411–1413, A8–9.

39. Mathur A, Roubin GS, Gomez CR, Iyer SS, Wong PM, Piamsomboon C, Yadav SS, Dean LS, Vitek JJ. Elective carotid artery stenting in the presence of contralateral occlusion. Am J Cardiol 1998; 81:1315–1317.

40. Al-Mubarak N, Roubin GS, Liu MW, Iyer SS, Dean LS, Vitek JJ. Late luminal loss following carotid artery stenting. Cathet Cardiovasc Intervent 1999; May:120.

41. Wang JS, Lai ST, Yu TJ, Weng ZC, Chang Y, Hwang JH. Synchronous carotid endarterectomy and myocardial revascularization. Chung Hua I Hsueh Tsa Chih (Taipei) 1994; 54:14–19.

42. Ohki T, Marin ML, Lyon RT, Berdejo GL, Soundararajan K, Ohki M, Yuan JG, Faries PL, Wain RA, Sanchez LA, Suggs WD, Veith FJ. Ex vivo human carotid artery bifurcation

stenting: correlation of lesion characteristics with embolic potential. J Vasc Surg 1998; 27:463–471.

43. Theron JG. Protected Angioplasty and Stenting of Atherosclerotic Stenosis at the Carotid Artery Bifurcation. Philadelphia: WB Saunders Co., 1998:466–473.

44. Vitek JJ, Raymon BC, Oh SJ. Innominate artery angioplasty. Am J Neuroradiol 1984; 5:113–114.

45. Vitek JJ. Subclavian artery angioplasty and the origin of the vertebral artery. Radiology 1989; 170:407–409.

46. Theron J. [Protected carotid angioplasty and carotid stents]. J Mal Vasc 1996; 21(suppl A):113–122.

47. Brown MM, Venables G, Clifton A, Gaines P, Taylor RS. Carotid endarterectomy vs carotid angioplasty. Lancet 1997; 349:880–881.

48. Hobson RW, 2nd, Brott T, Ferguson R, Roubin G, Moore W, Kuntz R, Howard G, Ferguson J. CREST: carotid revascularization endarterectomy versus stent trial. Cardiovasc Surg 1997; 5:457–458.

49. Al-Mubarak N, Roubin GS, Hobson RW, 2d, Ferguson R, Brott T, Moore W. Credentialing of stent operators for the Carotid Revascularization Endarterectomy vs. Stenting Trial "CREST." Stroke 2000; 73:97.

14

Current Benchmarks and Future Goals in Carotid Angioplasty and Stenting

Walter A. Tan, Chester R. Jarmolowski, Gustav R. Eles, and Mark H. Wholey
Pittsburgh Vascular Institute, University of Pittsburgh Medical Center–Shadyside Hospital, Pittsburgh, Pennsylvania

Michael H. Wholey
University of Texas Health Science Center at San Antonic, San Antonio, Texas

I. EXPERIENCE WITH PALMAZ STENTING IN CAROTID ARTERY STENOSIS AT THE PITTSBURGH VASCULAR INSTITUTE

Five stents are available for percutaneous carotid interventions at the Pittsburgh Vascular Institute (PVI). These include the self-expandable stents: the Wallstent (Schneider AG, Zurich, Switzerland), the SMART stent (Cordis Johnson & Johnson Interventional Systems, Warren, NJ), the Acculink stent (Guidant, Santa Clara, CA), and the newly developed Endotex stent (Endotex, Cupertino, CA). The other major category is the hand-mounted bare stents, in particular the slotted-tube (Palmaz) stent (Cordis, Warren, NJ). Until recently, our most extensive experience has been with the latter, which we describe here.

A. Study Population

Between April 1994 and February 1999, 285 patients underwent Palmaz stenting in 306 carotid arteries. In 12 cases only percutaneous transluminal angioplasty (PTA) was done, and these were analyzed by an intention-to-stent method. Fifty-six percent of this cohort was male. The mean age was 70.5 years, with an age range of 27–89 years. Of note, more than a third had coronary artery disease, and close to 40% were diabetic. Prior carotid endarterectomy had been performed in 35% of these patients.

A total of 159 patients (56%) were symptomatic, including 78 patients with stroke, 71 patients who presented with transient ischemic attacks (TIAs), and 14 with amaurosis fugax or monocular blindness (some patients had both a TIA and stroke). Of these symptomatic patients, 134 (84%) would not have met North American Symptomatic Carotid Endarterectomy Trial (NASCET) inclusion criteria (1). Similarly, 75 (59%) patients in the asymptomatic group would not have been eligible for the Asymptomatic Carotid Atherosclerosis trial (ACAS) (8).

B. Technique

Our procedural technique in the past with Palmaz stenting consisted of standard retrograde access via a common femoral artery with a 9-French vascular sheath. A 0.035-in. torquable guidewire in a 5-French diagnostic catheter is used to gain purchase into the external carotid artery. This is then switched to a 0.035-in. exchange length (260 cm) superstiff Amplatz wire (Medi-Tech, Natick, MA). A 7-French introducer (DVI, Temecula, CA) within a 9-French 90-cm guiding catheter (Brite-tip, Cordis Corp., Miami, FL) is employed coaxially and carefully advanced into the common carotid artery approximately 1 cm caudal to the carotid bifurcation. A 0.014-in. coronary extrasupport guidewire is then carefully advanced across the lesion with the distal tip placed in the cervical carotid artery at the level of the C2 vertebral body (4).

A 4.0 × 20 mm PTCA balloon catheter is typically used to predilate the lesion at 12–14 atmospheres (ATM). A Palmaz stent is selected based on lesion location and reference vessel dimensions and mounted by hand on a 120-cm, 0.018-in. guidewire-compatible balloon catheter (Jupiter, Cordis Corp., Miami, FL). The stent-balloon assembly is then advanced across the lesion and deployed using a single balloon inflation for 10 sec with 15 ATM.

All patients were pretreated with aspirin (325 mg daily) or ticlopidine (250 mg orally twice daily) for 5 days prior to the procedure.

Post procedure, patients were maintained on a regimen of aspirin 82 mg every day, and ticlopidine 500 mg daily for a week and 250 mg every day for 2 more weeks, or alternatively clopidogrel 75 mg daily for 3 weeks.

C. Results

There were eight technical failures for a technical success rate of 97.4%. Six of the eight technical failures resulted from unsatisfactory carotid artery access with the guide catheter. The other two failures resulted from complications during the procedure: one patient had a major stroke during diagnostic catheter manipulation, and one patient had severe seizures during balloon predilatation.

Thirty-day mortality was three (1.1%): one due to a major stroke, one due to pneumonia, and the third a Jehovah's witness who hemorrhaged during surgery for femoral artery pseudoaneurysm and refused transfusions. Neurological complications included three (1.1%) major and five (1.8%) minor strokes. A minor stroke was defined as a new neurological deficit that either resolved completely within 7 days or increased the NIH Stroke Scale by 3 or less. A major stroke was defined as a new neurological deficit that persisted after 7 days and increased the NIH Stroke Scale by 4 or more (9). Three (1.1%) patients had femoral artery pseudoaneurysms requiring surgical management. Three patients (1.1%) had long-term stent deformation, two of whom underwent successful reintervention.

II. OPTIMIZING OUTCOMES IN CBAS

The critical elements of effective and safe carotid stenting are delivery system profile, stent design, and distal emboli protection.

A. The Ideal Stent Design

The 3.8% stroke and death rate described in this series compares favorably to surgical outcomes reported in NASCET and other randomized clinical trials (1). Other groups such as Henry's have reported similarly low neurological complication rates (7). Of note, we have not been able to replicate these good results with the current generation of self-expanding stents. Hence, the results from Palmaz stenting of carotid artery disease still serve as logical benchmarks for newer stent designs. The main advantages of the Palmaz stent are low profile, and predictable and precise placement by balloon expansion (Table 1, Fig. 1). As opposed to the currently available self-expanding stents, these properties have allowed us to:

1. Use parsimonious stent lengths
2. Avoid stenting across the external carotid artery
3. Track smaller-caliber equipment across diseased extracranial vessel walls
4. Minimize translesional stent manipulation (adjustments forward and backward across the lesion)
5. Have shorter procedural time

The lower profile of the balloon shaft upon which this stent is mounted (Ranger or Jupiter balloons) means less traction, perturbation, and device "dottering" across diseased endothelial beds in the aortic arch and common carotid artery on the way to accessing the lesion. Added to this, the technically superior ease of positioning of the Palmaz-type stents (as opposed to self-expanding stents) may translate to less aortic arch and carotid artery trauma, thereby lowering procedural embolic risk. Minimal vessel trauma and parsimonious stenting may also yield lower rates of restenosis.

Table 1 Comparison of Carotid Stent Device Profiles: Outer-Diameter Measurements

Stent	Type	Approximate lesion crossing profile (F)	Minimum guide catheter size (F)
Palmaz	Balloon expandable	5.5	8
Wall	Self-expanding	7	9
Smart	Self-expanding	7	9
Acculink	Self-expanding	6	8
Endotex	Self-expanding	5	7

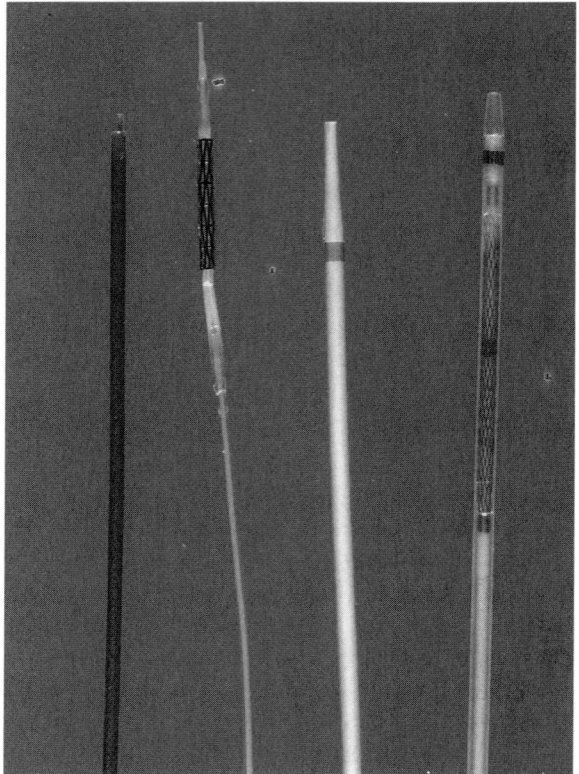

Figure 1 Visual comparison of carotid stent and delivery system profiles. (left to right) Endotex stent, Palmaz stent mounted on Ranger balloon, SMART stent, and Wall stent.

The major drawback of balloon-mounted stents is stent deformation or crushing from external compression. Reports of this phenomenon have been as high as 7–11% and have shifted clinical practice to the use of self-expanding stents (10–12). However, the superiority of these newer systems has yet to be proven (13), and further technological refinement is needed to match the desirable properties of balloon-mounted stents.

The ideal stent of the future should therefore have the following properties:

1. Low overall device (stent and delivery system) profile (Fig. 1)
2. Conformability to vessel contour (Fig. 2)
3. Precision deployment
4. Good radial force that can resist external compressive forces
5. Recrossability (edge control)

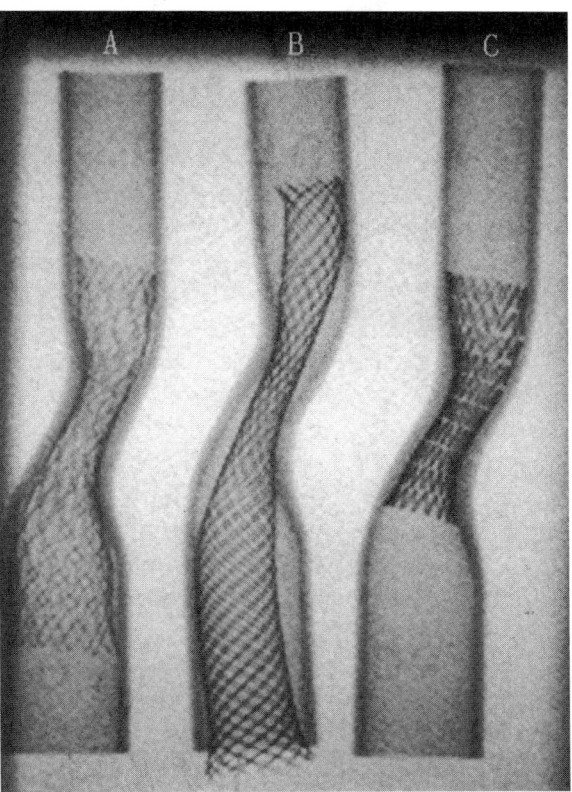

Figure 2 Stent conformability: ex vivo comparison within glass cylinders. (A) Endotex stent. (B) Wall stent. (C) SMART stent.

6. Trackable even through tortuous or calcified segments
7. Minimal cell size for better lesion coverage and to decrease the amount of plaque prolapse
8. Availability of wide selection of diameters and lengths (minimize stent-to-lesion ratio)
9. Tapering effect
10. Allowance for true bifurcation lesions (significant ostial disease in the external carotid artery)

B. Other Innovations for the Future

The stroke rate from diagnostic catheterization alone in NASCET was close to 1% (1), thus highlighting the fact that the aortic arch and proximal extracranial vessels carry a risk for embolic stroke that is independent from the target lesion (14–16). Therefore, ultimately, guide catheters should be developed that can selectively cannulate the left carotid and the innominate arteries with minimal manipulation, and at the same time provide adequate support without need for vessel intubation beyond the origins of common carotid arteries. Unlike the current state of mixing and matching separate components, equipment for CBAS should be developed as an entire dedicated system (wire, diagnostic catheter, guide, stent, and perhaps distal protection device) with a design specific to the configurations of the carotid arterial tree. This system should be miniaturized to allow the entire procedure to be performed over a 0.014-in. wire and aiming for a 5F delivery stent.

Furthermore, the refinement of distal emboli protection devices is a significant development toward decreasing the hazard for stroke periprocedurally (17). The ideal filter device should have a <3F profile on a 0.014-in. wire platform with good torque and tracking properties to negotiate all complex lesions atraumatically. It should also have good capture efficiency (for particles as small as 75–150 μ) and yet allow concomitant cerebral perfusion. The general categories are filters, balloon occluders, and circulatory control

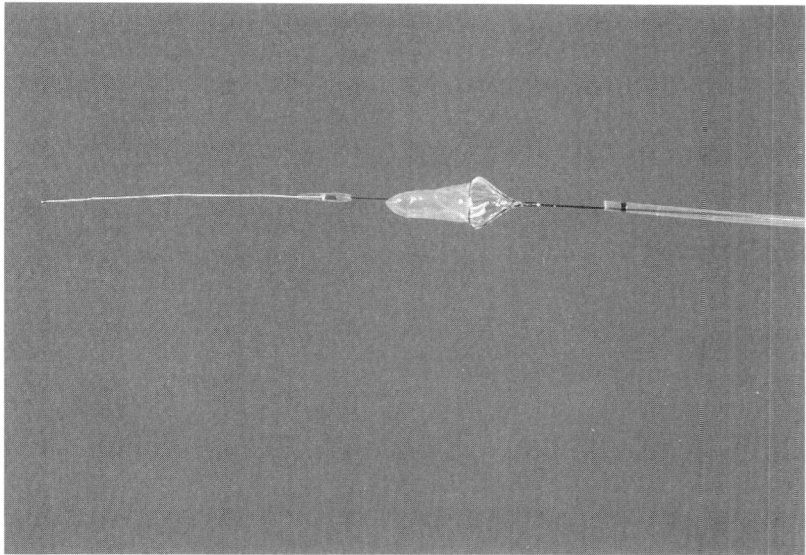

Figure 3 The EPI FilterWire (not FDA-approved), a low-profile porous filter-on-wire-type device with an adjustable nitinol frame to conform to vessel diameters between 3 and 7 mm.

devices, and are discussed elsewhere in this book (18,19). One example of such a device is depicted in Figure 3.

The glycoprotein IIb/IIIa receptor blocking agents may play only a supplementary role, as platelet emboli in the presence of adequate intraprocedural anticoagulation and perfusion pressure may constitute only a small proportion of total embolic events in CBAS.

III. REEXAMINING PATHOPHYSIOLOGICAL ASSUMPTIONS

Modern neuroimaging techniques can easily discern intra-cerebral hemorrhage from ischemic stroke, but it is still difficult to judge whether a significant carotid stenosis is the culprit by way of emboli or due to hemodynamic compromise. Twenty-eight percent of strokes in the NINDS Stroke Data Bank were of undetermined cause, while only 6% were attributed to large-artery occlusion (20,21). Emboli from mild lesions or irregularities not fulfilling standard criteria for significant obstruction conceivably can account for some of these cryptogenic strokes. Indirect evidence for this is embolic phenomena in spite of known chronic occlusion of ipsilateral carotid arteries, or in the context of mild but ulcerated lesions where flow insufficiency is not an issue (22). In fact, in contrast to the proven efficacy of bypasses for coronary ischemia, extracranial to intracranial (EC/IC) may have failed because of failure to prevent embolic phenomena (23). Vessel flow is certainly not everything (24). Careful investigations by Powers and colleagues have found no correlation between neurological events and hemodynamically significant carotid lesions proven by positron emission tomography (PET) measurements of regional cerebral blood flow (rCBF) and blood volume (rCBV) (25). In addition, in a retrospective study they performed, there were three ipsilateral strokes at 1-year postdischarge after EC/IC bypass in 21 patients with proven hemodynamic compromise, as opposed to none in a matched group of 23 nonsurgical patients (26). This was in spite of improved cerebral hemodynamics after bypass (27).

Therefore, while interventionalists typically focus on reestablishing unrestricted flow by means of dilating the diseased carotid artery to adequate dimensions, the true mechanism of benefit may be the attenuation of artery-to-artery embolization. With stenting, lesion quiescence is attained via lesion coverage, plaque sealing, and stabilization by fibrosis. The implications of this may not be trivial: if this proves to be true, interventionalists must learn to be content with lesion coverage without balloon postdilatation even with an "apparently" significant residual stenosis (28), as long as the lumen is above a certain minimal lesional diameter (MLD) cutoff, especially with the self-expanding stents. The ultimate goal becomes a near-zero tolerance for complications (the large majority of which occur intra-procedurally), and aiming to achieve *maximal plaque sealing* with *minimal plaque perturbation*.

IV. SUMMARY AND CONCLUSIONS

Several randomized clinical trials have established the efficacy of endarterectomy for the prevention of stroke from carotid artery stenosis (1,2). The accumulated observational data and one randomized clinical trial suggest comparable benefit-to-risk ratio with percutaneous methods (3–7). While newer self-expanding stents address the problem of external stent compression, the balloon-expandable, slotted-tube stent remains the benchmark with regard to clinical outcome. This is related to its long history of widespread use, its low profile, and the capability for precise implantation. These features translate to parsimonious stent length requirements, less catheter manipulation, and shorter procedural time. These may have clinical impact with respect to lower embolic risk, avoidance of stenting across arterial branches, shorter stent lengths, and perhaps even less restenosis. Important directions for the development of optimal equipment for carotid stenting are outlined.

Furthermore, a reexamination of underlying therapeutic tenets may be in order. Plaque sealing and stabilization by fibrosis may be a more important mechanism for stroke prevention than relief of hemodynamic obstruction. These concepts hold critical implications for the development of devices and drug strategies that might improve procedural and clinical outcomes.

ACKNOWLEDGMENTS

The authors would like to express their gratitude to Rosann Bost for her superb secretarial assistance, and to David L. Stebbins for photographic work.

REFERENCES

1. North American Symptomatic Carotid Endarterectomy Trial Collaborators. Beneficial effect of carotid endarterectomy in symptomatic patients with high-grade carotid stenosis. N Engl J Med 1991; 325(7):445–453.
2. Randomised trial of endarterectomy for recently symptomatic carotid stenosis: final results of the MRC European Carotid Surgery Trial (ECST). Lancet 1998; 351(9113): 1379–1387.
3. Sivaguru A, et al. European carotid angioplasty trial. Endovasc Surg 1996; 3(1):16–20.
4. Wholey MH, et al. Endovascular stents for carotid artery occlusive disease. J Endovasc Surg 1997; 4(4):326–338.
5. Roubin GS, et al. Carotid stent-supported angioplasty: a neurovascular intervention to prevent stroke. Am J Cardiol 1996; 78(3A):8–12.
6. Wholey MH, et al. Current global status of carotid artery stent placement. Cathet Cardiovasc Diagn 1998; 44(1):1–6.
7. Henry M, et al. Angioplasty and stenting of the extracranial carotid arteries. J Endovasc Surg 1998; 5(4):293–304.
8. Asymptomatic Carotid Atherosclerosis Study Group. Study design for randomized prospective trial of carotid endarterectomy for asymptomatic atherosclerosis. Stroke 1989; 20(7):844–849.
9. Brott T, et al. Measurements of acute cerebral infarction: a clinical examination scale. Stroke 1989; 20(7):864–870.
10. Yadav JS, et al. Elective stenting of the extracranial carotid arteries. Circulation 1997; 95(2):376–381.
11. Mathur A, et al. Palmaz stent compression in patients following carotid artery stenting. Cathet Cardiovasc Diagn 1997; 41(2):137–140.
12. Wholey MH. Regarding "Stent deformation and intimal hy-

perplasia complicating treatment of a post-carotid endarterectomy intimal flap with a Palmaz stent." J Vasc Surg 1997; 26(5):897–899.

13. Naylor AR, et al. Randomized study of carotid angioplasty and stenting versus carotid endarterectomy: a stopped trial. J Vasc Surg 1998; 28(2):326–334.

14. Amarenco P, Cohen A. [Atherosclerosis of the aortic arch: a possible new source of cerebral embolism.] Ann Cardiol Angeiol (Paris) 1994; 43(5):278–281.

15. Amarenco P, et al. The prevalence of ulcerated plaques in the aortic arch in patients with stroke. N Engl J Med 1992; 326(4):221–225.

16. Davies KN, Humphrey PR. Complications of cerebral angiography in patients with symptomatic carotid territory ischaemia screened by carotid ultrasound. J Neurol Neurosurg Psychiatry 1993; 56(9):967–972.

17. Ohki T, et al., Ex vivo human carotid artery bifurcation stenting: correlation of lesion characteristics with embolic potential. J Vasc Surg 1998; 27(3):463–471.

18. Theron J, et al., New triple coaxial catheter system for carotid angioplasty with cerebral protection. Am J Neuroradiol 1990; 11(5):869–874.

19. Theron J. [Protected carotid angioplasty and carotid stents.] J Mal Vasc 1996; 21(suppl A):113–122.

20. Foulkes MA, et al., The Stroke Data Bank; design, methods, and baseline characteristics. Stroke 1988; 19(5):547–554.

21. Sacco RL, et al. Infarcts of undetermined cause: the NINCDS Stroke Data Bank. Ann Neurol 1989; 25(4):382–390.

22. Eliasziw M, et al. Significance of plaque ulceration in symptomatic patients with high-grade carotid stenosis. North American Symptomatic Carotid Endarterectomy Trial. Stroke 1994; 25(2):304–308.

23. EC/IC Bypass Study Group. Failure of extracranial-intracranial arterial bypass to reduce the risk of ischemic stroke. Results of an international randomized trial. N Engl J Med 1985; 313(19):1191–1200.

24. Tan WA, Moliterno DJ. TIMI flow and surrogate end points: what you see is not always what you get. Am Heart J 1998; 136(4 pt 1):570–573.

25. Powers WJ, Tempe LW, Grubb RL Jr. Influence of cerebral

hemodynamics on stroke risk: one-year follow-up of 30 medically treated patients. Ann Neurol 1989; 25(4):325–330.

26. Powers WJ, Grubb RL Jr, Raichle ME. Clinical results of extracranial-intracranial bypass surgery in patients with hemodynamic cerebrovascular disease. J Neurosurg 1989; 70(1):61–67.

27. Schmiedek P. EC-IC bypass in hemodynamic cerebrovascular disease. J Neurosurg 1989; 71(3):464–466.

28. Crawley F, et al. Delayed improvement in carotid artery diameter after carotid angioplasty. Stroke 1997; 28(3):574–579.

15

Treatment of Carotid Atherosclerotic Disease

Carotid Endarterectomy or Stenting?

Jay S. Yadav
The Cleveland Clinic Foundation, Cleveland, Ohio

There are estimated to be over 700,000 strokes per year in the United States alone and stroke remains a major public health problem in the industrialized countries. A significant proportion of strokes are caused by extracranial carotid atherosclerotic disease. As the population ages, the incidence of stroke and carotid disease will continue to increase. As we need to care for ever more elderly and frail patients with multiple comorbid conditions, it is imperative that we develop less invasive endovascular alternatives to traditional open surgical techniques. We will review the pros and cons of endarterectomy and stenting for carotid disease and the indications for each procedure on the basis of current evidence.

Carotid endarterectomy (CEA) is an excellent and well-established procedure with over a 40-year history, and in the past few years it has been validated by carefully performed randomized, controlled trials. Like all medical treatments, however, it does have some limitations. The limitations of CEA fall into the following areas: anatomical; cranial nerve palsies; selection bias in the randomized trials; worse results in unselected patients, and poor results in certain patient subsets with comorbid conditions.

Carotid disease most commonly occurs at the carotid bifurcation, which in most patients is located at the C3–4 vertebral interspace. In about 10% of patients, however, the carotid lesion is not easily accessible surgically (1). The bifurcation itself can be shifted superiorly so that mandibular dislocation is required to reach it. The lesion may not occur at the bifurcation or may occur in tandem with a bifurcation lesion with the most common other sites being the carotid siphon and the innominate or left common carotid ostia. Patients who have previously had radical neck dissection for carcinoma often develop carotid disease due to their heavy smoking histories and these patients are poor candidates for endarterectomy due to their extensive scarring. Cervical radiation therapy either alone or in combination with radical neck dissection also makes endarterectomy quite challenging and difficult. Other anatomical problems include the presence of a tracheostomy, burns with or without skin grafting, severe cervical arthritis, previous cervical spine fusion, and severe obesity. Given the complexity and morbidity of the surgical approaches for these anatomical situations, endovascular techniques have become the treatment of choice for patients with them at many major medical centers.

Cranial nerve palsies generally occur due to retraction injury to the nerves during neck dissection and exposure of the carotid artery. The most commonly involved cranial nerves include the hypoglossal, recurrent laryngeal, and branches of the trigeminal nerve. The most common symptoms are dysarthria, dysphagia, dysphonia, and lower face and neck numbness or paresthesia. The incidence varies from 7.5% in the North American Symptomatic Carotid Endarterectomy Trial (NASCET) to 27% in some series (2). Cranial nerve palsies may take several weeks to resolve and may occasionally be permanent. Bilateral cranial nerve palsies can be quite disabling leading to severe dysarthria or dysphonia and sufficiently severe dysphagia to require a feeding tube. A patient with a major preexisting cranial nerve palsy who has developed contralateral carotid stenosis is a poor CEA candidate owing to the risk of bilateral cranial nerve palsies.

There have been several randomized trials of CEA versus medical treatment with the North American Symptomatic Carotid Endarterecomy Trial (NASCET) and Asymptomatic Carotid Atherosclerosis Study (ACAS) being the definitive trials for symptomatic and asymptomatic disease, respectively (2,3). Both trials had multiple exclusion criteria that were similar. Reasons for exclusion included: age greater than 79 years, comorbidity likely to cause death in 5 years, severe cardiac disease; atrial fibrillation; severe lung disease, uncontrolled hypertension, uncontrolled diabetes, unstable angina, or myocardial infarction within 6 months. To qualify for NASCET, surgeons had to perform more than 25 CEAs per year and have a less than 6% per year stroke rate in symptomatic patients. Importantly, only one-third of the patients having endarterectomies at the trial hospitals were enrolled into NASCET. The reasons why these patients were not enrolled and their outcomes were not recorded. Similarly, in ACAS only one out of every 25 patients screened were enrolled. Therefore, there has been great concern about patient selection bias in these trials and the applicability of these results to the general patient population. These concerns were confirmed by a recent review of carotid endartectomy mortality in Medicare patients. Wennberg et al. reviewed the 113,000 Medicare patients who had CEAs at trial (NASCET, ACAS) and nontrial hospitals during 1992 and 1993. At the trial hospitals, the overall mortality was 1.4% while at nontrial hospitals, it was 1.7% and at low-volume hospitals, it was 2.5%. The mortality in NASCET was 0.6% and in ACAS it was 0.1% (4). So in the same hospitals that participated in NASCET and ACAS, the mortality for patients not in the trial was at least threefold higher suggesting that a low-risk subset of patients was randomized in the trials.

Further evidence that the surgical complication rates are substantially higher outside of the randomized trials comes from a retrospective chart review of all CEAs performed at 12 major academic medical centers by McCrory et al. (5). In 1160 patients the risk of stroke, myocardial infarction (MI), or death was 6.9%. In patients who were symptomatic the risk was 9.5%; in patients over age 75 the risk was 11.8%; in patients with angina the risk was 9.9% and in patients going on to coronary artery bypass (CABG) during the same hospitalization the risk was 40%. Moreover, the retrospective chart review methodology of this study may underestimate the true incidence of complications.

It is commonly stated that NASCET is already outdated and the current surgical complication rates are much lower. Data do not support this viewpoint. In a comprehensive meta-analysis of all CEA articles published until 1996,

Rothwell et al. found that the incidence of stroke and death was 4.34% from 1980 to 1984, 5.28% from 1985 to 1989, and 6.08% from 1990 to 1994 (6). Furthermore, they found that the incidence of complications was directly related to the precision of the neurological examination: in series that had only a surgical author the complication rate was 2.3% while series with a neurologist had a complication rate of 7.7%. They also note a useful method for checking the accuracy of reported data. In natural history studies of stroke it has been found that the case fatality ratio for stroke is 10–20% meaning that in patients having a stroke one or two out of 10 will die. This has been borne out in the randomized endarterectomy trials with NASCET having a stroke case fatality of 17% and ECST with a stroke case fatality ratio of 13%. Therefore, if a surgical series is reported with a mortality rate of 1% and a stroke rate of 1% giving a stroke case fatality ratio of 50%, it is possible that the minor strokes are not being captured.

Restenosis occurs in 5–20% of CEA patients depending upon the definition used and the duration of follow-up. Due to the scarring from the previous surgery and the lack of a clearly defined media-adventitia border, the complication rates for reoperations are considerably higher, ranging from 7% to 10% at major institutions, and the AHA guidelines for endarterectomy consider a 10% complication rate acceptable (7). Since carotid stenting is not affected by the scar tissue, it appears to be particularly well suited for this group of patients. In the first reported experience with restenotic lesions, we found carotid stenting to have a complication rate of 4%.

In NASCET, patients with contralateral carotid occlusions had an almost threefold higher complication rate of 14.3% compared to patients without contralateral occlusions. We have reported on our initial series of 31 patients with contralateral occlusions treated with carotid stenting with only a 3.2% complication rate (9). The very brief (15–30 sec) interruption of cerebral blood flow during carotid stenting as compared to CEA even when a shunt is used leads to much less cerebral ischemia in patients undergoing treatment in the presence of a contralateral occlusion.

Patients who present with synchronous coronary and carotid disease remain a management challenge even in the most expert surgical hands. Sequential or combined CEA and CABG is associated with high morbidity and mortality rates. A meta-analysis of 56 reports on combined CABG and CEA revealed a permanent stroke risk of 6.2%, a Q-wave MI risk of 4.7%, and a mortality of 5.6% (7). At the Cleveland Clinic, we currently often manage these patients with a carotid stent followed by CABG: 21 patients have now undergone successful CABG, and two patients have undergone successful heart transplantation without a stroke, MI, or death.

Some multicenter data are now available for carotid stenting. In a review of the major international carotid stenting centers, Wholey et al. found a complication rate of 5.6% in 2591 patients and a restenosis rate of less than 5% (10). Martin Brown (personal communication) has conducted a randomized trial of carotid endarterectomy versus carotid angioplasty with provisional stenting in the United Kingdom: 504 patients were randomized with 253 patients receiving surgery and 251 patients receiving angioplasty with 25% of the angioplasty patients receiving stents. The periprocedural complication rate was identical in both groups at 6.3%.

Although the results of carotid stenting and angioplasty are surprisingly good particularly in high risk patients, embolization remains an unsolved problem. Transcranial Doppler (TCD) monitoring of the middle cerebral artery during carotid stenting has shown subclinical embolization in all patients. Embolization appears to be the cause of all acute complications associated with carotid stenting since vessel closure is extremely rare. Both pharmacological and mechanical approaches are being tried to reduce the incidence of complications.

Platelet glycoprotein IIb/IIIa inhibition with abciximab has markedly reduced cardiac events after coronary balloon angioplasty. This experience has been applied to selected patients by Chastain and colleagues in 22 carotid stent procedures involving visible thrombus, total occlusion, or acute stroke (11). In their series of high-risk lesions, two (7%) central nervous system bleeding complications occurred: one a hemorrhagic transformation of a previously ischemic stroke and the other a subarachnoid hemorrhage from a ruptured aneurysm. The aneurysm was not initially visualized because of its location beyond a total occlusion, and this patient later died. Periprocedural glycoprotein IIb/IIIa receptor inhibition may be safer and more effective when used in a routine, prophylactic manner, and this approach is currently being evaluated at the Cleveland Clinic. We have now electively treated 95 patients with abciximab without periprocedural strokes or hemorrhage. One patient had a small hemorrhage into a previously infarcted area 4 days post procedure and made a good recovery.

Rather than a pharmacological approach, some investigators have employed mechanical means in an effort to reduce the incidence of stroke and embolization with carotid stenting. Henry and colleagues stented 27 carotid arteries using a prototype cerebral-protection balloon device and compared their results to 104 cases treated without the device (12). These are low-profile, balloon-tipped guidewires, designed to block cerebral emboli when positioned in the internal carotid artery beyond the lesion. The protection balloon occludes the runoff circulation to the brain, trapping any particles dislodged during balloon dilation or stent delivery so that they can be extracted via aspiration with a seperate specialized catheter. Henry and colleagues reported two major strokes with the cerebral protection balloon and one major stroke, one minor stroke, and three transient ischemic attacks without its use. In an effort to reduce the complication rates associated with balloon occlusion devices, filter devices that allow continued perfusion while capturing emboli also are being developed. Improved devices of this type, which should be available this year, have the potential for markedly lowering the incidence of stroke associated with carotid stenting.

Carotid angioplasty and stenting is still being performed with currently available devices not specifically designed for the procedure. This year we should have available guide catheters and stents specifically designed for the carotid circulation. Guide catheters that allow easy atraumatic access of the common carotid ostium and nitinol stents that deploy precisely with minimal shortening and have low-profile delivery systems will make the procedure easier, quicker, and safer.

In certain patient groups—those with contralateral occlusions, postendarterectomy restenosis, synchronous carotid and coronary disease, preexisting major cranial nerve palsies, very distal and very proximal lesions, and unusual cervical anatomy or scarring—carotid stenting currently represents a reasonable alternative to CEA. For the low-risk patient, CEA should remain the standard of care. Emboli prevention devices and nitinol stents will greatly expand the spectrum of carotid disease that can be safely treated with endovascular therapy.

REFERENCES

1. Huber P, ed. Krayenbuhl/Yasargil Cerebral Angiography. New York: Thieme, 1982: p. 37.
2. North American Symptomatic Carotid Endarterectomy Trial Collaborators. Beneficial effect of carotid endarterectomy in symptomatic patients with high-grade carotid stenosis. N Engl J Med 1991; 325:445–453.
3. Asymptomatic Carotid Atherosclerosis Study Group. Endarterectomy for asymptomatic carotid artery stenosis. JAMA 1995; 273:421–428.
4. Wennberg DE, Lucas FL, Birkmeyer JD, et al. Variation in

carotid endarterectomy mortality in the medicare population. Trial hospitals, volume and patient characteristics. JAMA 1998; 279:1278–1281.

5. McCrory DC, Goldstein LB, Samsa GP, et al. Predicting complications of carotid endarterectomy. Stroke 1993; 24:1285–1291.

6. Rothwell PM, Slattery J, Warlow CP. A systematic comparison of the risks of stroke and death due to carotid endarterectomy for symptomatic and asymptomatic stenosis. Stroke 1996; 27:266–269.

7. Moore WS, Barnett HJM, Beebe HG, et al. Guidelines for carotid endarterectomy. Circulation 1995; 91:566–579.

8. Gasecki AP, Eliasziv M, Ferguson GG, et al. Long term prognosis and effect of endarterectomy in patients with symptomatic severe carotid stenosis and contralateral carotid stenosis or occlusion: results from NASCET. J Neurosurg 1995; 83:778–782.

9. Mathur A, Roubin GS, Gomez CR, et al. Elective carotid artery stenting in the presence of contralateral occlusion. Am J Cardiol 1998; 81:1315–1317.

10. Wholey MH, Wholey M, Bergeron P, et al. Current global status of carotid artery stent placement. Cathet Cardiovasc Diagn 1998; 44:1–6.

11. Chastain HD II, Wong P, Mathur A, et al. Does abciximab reduce complications of cerebral vascular stenting in high risk lesions? Circulation 1997; 96(suppl I):1–283.

12. Henry M, Amor M, Henry I, et al. Endovascular treatment of atherosclerotic stenosis of the internal carotid. JVIR 1998; 9(suppl):162.

16

Current Status and Future Considerations in Carotid Bifurcation Angioplasty and Stenting

Max Amor
U.C.C.I. Polyclinique d'Essey, Essey-les-Nancy, France

James Robert Wilentz
Albert Einstein College of Medicine–Beth Israel Medical Center, New York, New York

Michel Henry
U.C.C.I. Polyclinique d'Essey, Essey-les-Nancy, France

I. INTRODUCTION

Carotid endovascular intervention has undergone significant evolution since its inception. There are now multiple routes for access, choices for guidewires, balloons, and stents, methods of protection against embolization, techniques for pre- and postprocedural evaluation, as well as new choices for concomitant medical therapy. As the contributors to this book make clear, there have emerged areas of consensus in therapy as well as areas of continued discussion and questioning. We will try to provide an overview of a field in rapid evolution.

II. PATHOPHYSIOLOGY AND PROCEDURAL GOALS

Atherosclerotic vascular disease leads to morbidity and mortality both by embolization and by diminution of blood flow. In the carotid circulation, the primary mode of morbidity is embolic rather than by hemodynamic disturbance, as opposed to that in most other vascular beds. As discussed by Tan et al. elsewhere in this book (1), when the etiology of stroke was sought in the 1273 stroke patients in the NINCDS Stroke Data Bank, 40% were found to be infarcts of undetermined cause (IUC). When only those 138 IUC patients who had both CT and angiographic evaluation were considered, the clinical syndrome and computed tomographic and angiographic findings in 91 (65.9%) of these 138 IUC cases were clearly not attributable to large-artery thrombosis and could permit reclassification of the infarct as due to some form of embolism, while only 31 cases (22.5%) could be reclassified as due to stenosis or thrombosis of a large artery (2). The inference is that both stroke and the recurrent symptom of transient ischemic attack attributable to carotid atherosclerosis are due in large part to embolization. Indeed, embolic stroke may occur in ulcerated lesions with only modest degrees of stenosis. These data as well as the finding that morbidity and mortality for symptomatic (embologenic) carotid disease is significantly higher than for asymptomatic (nonembologenic) carotid disease lead to the consideration that degree of stenosis, while of great importance in other vascular beds, may be less important in the cerebral circulation while passivation of active carotid plaques is likely of paramount import and should be considered a primary goal of carotid therapy. This has important implications both for the choice and placement of a carotid stent and for the indications for stenting of a carotid lesion.

When thinking about the goals for carotid interventional therapy, then, it must be borne in mind that reduction in percent diameter stenosis, while important, may miss the objective if the entire embologenic plaque is not covered. With coverage of the entire embologenic plaque, the potential exists for passivation of the disease by the mechanism of stent-induced plaque sealing and fibrosis of a previously active lipid-laden friable lesion.

III. HISTORY

The question of treatment choice for carotid arterial disease has generated multiple studies over time. Three landmark studies were the North American Symptomatic Carotid Endarterectomy Trial (NASCET) (3,4), the European Carotid Surgery Trial (ECST) (5), and the Endarterectomy for Asymptomatic Carotid Artery Stenosis trial (ACAS) (6). These studies clearly established the superiority of carotid endarterectomy over available medical therapy in symptomatic patients with a significant degree of carotid stenosis (>70%), and strongly suggested surgical superiority over medical therapy both in the symptomatic group with moderate stenosis (50–69%) and in the asymptomatic group with stenosis > 60%. Limitations of these studies are their low frequency of recruitment among women (70% men in NASCET) and the subsequent absence of finding of benefit of this therapy for women, as well as limitations shared by all large randomized trials such as inapplicability of inclusion/exclusion factors to real-world patients, a high degree of surgical expertise required to participate in the studies, differences in surgical mortality between participants in these studies, and contemporary nonstudy sites especially lower-volume institutions (7). In addition, the medical therapy used did not include clopidogrel, which has been shown subsequently to add to the effect of aspirin in diminishing subsequent vascular events in patients with cerebrovascular or coronary disease (8). These caveats aside, the superiority of carotid surgical intervention over medical therapy for significant symptomatic and asymptomatic stenosis has been firmly established.

IV. EMERGENCE OF PERCUTANEOUS INTERVENTION

Despite the excellent results of carotid endarterectomy, problems remained. In NASCET, the reported stroke morbidity and mortality rate was 6.7%, in ECST 7.5%. In other series of higher-risk patient subgroups, rates have varied with different reporting techniques, but have ranged from as low as 0–2% (9,10) to as high as 18% (11,12). Given the documented benefits of surgical treatment, the search for less invasive means to treat carotid stenosis led in the early 1980s to the emergence of carotid angioplasty (13–16) and in the mid-1990s to the introduction of carotid stenting (17–22). At the outset, the role of carotid angioplasty and stenting was explored for patient subgroups felt to be at higher risk for CEA (Table 1).

Three randomized trials of carotid endarterectomy versus stenting have been undertaken. The results of the European Carotid and Vertebral Transluminal Angioplasty

Table 1 High-Risk Groups for Carotid Endarterectomy/
NASCET Exclusions

High-risk local surgical anatomy	Previous radical neck dissection
	Previous radiation therapy
	Surgically inaccessible
	Stenosis site supramandibular (high bifurcation, high lesion)
	"Rigid" neck
	Restenosis of previous CEA
	Disease at the origin CCA[a]
Other cerebro-vascular disease	Contralateral carotid occlusion[a]
	Concomitant vertebral occlusions [assessment of circle of Willis)[a]
	Concomitant significant intracranial tandem carotid stenosis
	Previous functionally limiting ipsilateral infarct
Comorbidity	?Advanced age > 80[b,c]
	?Atrial fibrillation[b]
	?Cancer with life expectancy < 5 years[b]
	Renal failure
	Pulmonary insufficiency
	Diabetes mellitus
	Recent stroke or unstable neurological syndrome
	Unstable angina, recent MI, heart failure, respiratory failure

[a] Not a NASCET exclusion but surgically high risk.
[b] NASCET exclusion but without demonstrated increase in surgical risk.
[c] Originally excluded but allowed in NASCET continuation.

Study (CAVATAS) (23,24) trial will be reported later this year comparing surgery and angioplasty for both carotid and vertebral stenoses. The early results of the study, published in Britain in 1999 (25), and presented orally at the AHA International Stroke meeting in 1999, suggest a similar disabling stroke and death rate of 6.3% for CEA and 6.4% for interventional procedures. Another early trial in

Britain was stopped because of a higher-than-expected rate of complications in the stent cohort (26). A trial with the Schneider Wallstent was also stopped because of poor recruitment (27). Despite very encouraging results from the nonrandomized series, there is a dearth of data with which to compare carotid stenting with surgical therapy. However, two ongoing trials, CREST and CASET (28,29), and more recent data on carotid stenting will yield further insight on the future potential of carotid stenting especially with measures taken to protect the brain parenchyma.

V. METHODS OF CAROTID INTERVENTION

A. Preprocedural Evaluation

Prior to contemplating an intervention in the carotid bifurcation, the team must have a disciplined method in place for complete evaluation of the patient, the lesion, and the brain parenchyma. It is essential to have not only excellent preprocedural angiographic information, but also high-quality ultrasound imaging, fast CT, or MRA vascular and parenchymal imaging. Without knowledge of the status of the other major cerebral perfusion vessels (contralateral carotid, vertebrals), course of collaterals if present (ECA-ICA), status of the circle of Willis, presence of other carotid or intracerebral arterial stenoses and aneurysms, location and extent of previous cerebral infarctions, it is impossible to understand the degree of risk of the procedure at each point and to map out the most effective and least risky way to proceed. An occlusive protection technique that may work perfectly in a patient with open contralateral carotid and vertebral vessels will likely be very poorly tolerated in a patient without other sources of cerebral perfusion. A protection device that relies on reversal of flow and flushing of debris into the ECA may prove disastrous in the presence of important ECA-ICA collaterals. A patient with previous extensive contralateral infarction will be much more vul-

nerable to the effects of embolization from the carotid treatment site. Moreover, the effects of carotid dilatation and
restoration of the forward pressure head in a patient with
a recent ipsilateral infarction are unpredictable and may
lead to hyperemia and hemorrhagic transformation of the
infarct. A tandem stenosis higher in the ipsilateral ICA, if
severe and untreated, may annul the effect of bifurcation
treatment, or may provide a site for wire dissection or en-
trapment of embolic debris. Undetected intracerebral aneurysm may also provide a site for slow or rapid and cata-
strophic bleeding. Sophisticated neuro "rescue" techniques
such as intracerebral catheter placements for thrombo-
aspiration/disruption/local lysis and intracerebral stent
placement for occlusive dissection should be available to
the operator for optimal patient safety.

Parenchymography in two projections prior to and
after the carotid intervention is extremely helpful in immediate evaluation of cerebral blood flow and in recognition of
any acute adverse effect on cerebral flow after intervention.
This may also be particularly helpful in distinguishing intraprocedural embolism from contrast-induced encephalopathy.

It goes without saying that a careful clinical evaluation
highlighting the degree of activity of disease in each vascular bed, especially in the case of the multivascular patient,
must be performed prior to the intervention and must be
borne in mind by the interventional team at the time of therapy. The patient with crescendo TIAs and moderate coronary disease with effort angina only should have the carotid
lesion treated first. Similarly, the patient with crescendo
angina, a 95% LAD stenosis, and an asymptomatic 75%
ICA lesion should probably have the LAD treated first. The
patient with unstable angina and clear-cut surgical coronary anatomy (left main CAD, severe three-vessel disease
with lesions inimical to coronary angioplasty) as well as a
significant carotid stenosis should be stabilized medically
as much as possible and then quickly treated with carotid

intervention followed by planned coronary surgery the following day or later in the same hospital stay.

B. Periprocedural Medical Treatment

All patients should be prepared with clopidogrel (ticlopidine should probably be abandoned owing to increased prevalence of thrombotic thrombocytopenic purpura and neutropenia) and ASA, and atropine should be given prior to bifurcation dilatation, except in the case of severe three-vessel or left main coronary patients who are better managed by preangioplasty temporary transvenous pacemaker insertion. This maneuver avoids the tachycardia and ischemia that may accompany an effective dose of atropine used to prevent severe vagally mediated bradycardia during carotid dilatation. The doses of chronically administered antihypertensive drugs should be reduced, and beta blockers withheld prior to the procedure since atropine may be ineffective in the presence of therapeutic beta blockade. In addition, beta blockade may worsen the occasional prolonged significant hypotension that may accompany bifurcation dilatation, and may increase the need for adrenergic infusion support. Heparin is given in conventional doses, and more recently, platelet glycoprotein IIB-IIIA inhibitors have been investigated as adjuncts to carotid stenting (30,31).

C. Access

There are three potential approaches into the vascular system for carotid intervention: femoral, brachial, and direct puncture into the common carotid (Table 2). Currently the femoral approach is the most commonly used, allowing excellent guide support via an 8 or 9F 90-cm multipurpose guide placed in the common carotid over a .035-in. wire directed toward or anchored in the external carotid. This can be done either directly, or, in cases of difficult angulation and access, by placement of a Simmons, Vitek, Head-

Table 2 Access Choices for Carotid Intervention

	Femoral	Brachial	Direct puncture
Advantages	Choice of large guide or sheath for large device and excellent support. Entry site easily compressible and remote from treatment site.	Useful for difficult access, aortoiliac disease; avoids aortic debris; radial approach may be used with rapid ambulation. Entry site easily compressible and remote from treatment site.	Alternative that does not require complex catheterization skills, may be appealing to vascular surgeon; extravascular closure device.
Disadvantages	Access may be difficult, especially in patients with multifocal vascular disease and aortoiliac disease.	Guide size limited. Guide support limited due to arch angulation and necessity to traverse arch to contralateral vessel.	Entry site not easily compressible and close to treatment site. Consequences of local bleeding or arterial trauma more severe.

hunter, or other diagnostic catheter into the common carotid, followed by placement of the .035-in. hydrophilic wire into the external carotid, advancement of the diagnostic catheter into the external, and exchange of the wire for an "extrastiff" .035-in. 300-cm guidewire, over which the guide catheter is then placed into the common carotid just below the bifurcation (32). The usefulness of the hydrophilic wire cannot be overstated. With careful attention to keeping these wires properly wet and flushed, they offer a highly lubricious crossing profile while retaining good torquability.

From the femoral approach, two types of conduit have been used, a 90-cm braided 7F sheath introducer or a 90-cm multipurpose or angled 8 or 9F guiding catheter. The advantage of the sheath is the larger inner diameter with a smaller puncture size, but this is traded off for a less- or nonmanipulable conduit with poorer support than the guiding catheter. The sheath method also may require the extra step of replacing the dilator when recrossing the stent, and this may make urgent reaccess to the ICA distal to the stent much more difficult if neurorescue or distal stenting is required to repair dissection (Table 3). In addition, a nonguided approach is possible (though rarely used) as with other peripheral angioplasty, where after diagnostic angiography and road mapping, an angioplasty guidewire is placed through the diagnostic catheter in the common carotid, after which the diagnostic catheter is exchanged for the treatment balloon, which is passed into the lesion using the road map from the diagnostic angiogram. Position may be confirmed by passage of a pigtail catheter and use of subtraction angiography. After treatment, results may be confirmed by angiography using the guiding system, the balloon, or the pigtail (33). The choice of approach for access to the carotid bifurcation stenosis is dictated in part by operator preference but principally by patient arterial characteristics. In the presence of significant aortoiliac disease, approaches other than the femoral are desired. In

Table 3 Choice of Conduit for Carotid Bifurcation Angioplasty and Stenting

	Guide	Sheath
Size	8–9F	7F
Length	90–100 cm	90 cm
Supports large device	++	+++
Maneuverability from aorta to CCA	++	+++
Direction of guidewire from CCA to ICA	+++	–
Balloon and stent passage	++	+++
Recrossing the stent	Easy (can bring guide forward during balloon deflation)	Difficult (may have to replace dilator)
Visualization	++	++
Avoidance of air bubbles	++	+

these cases, either the brachial or the direct common carotid approach described by Bergeron and Diethrich and their groups elsewhere in this book may provide an alternative route (34,35).

D. Guidewires

Although the majority of interventions in the peripheral arteries are performed using balloons requiring .035-in. wires, in the carotid arteries, the risks of embolization posed by the use of large balloons, the large size of the guide catheter required, and the ability to use the smaller coronary system militates against their use in this setting. We have chosen to use the .014- or .018-in. wire systems with coronary-type balloon catheters as will be described later. One variant of this technique is to leave the .035-in. wire in place in the external carotid to enhance the stability of the guiding catheter in cases where the arterial anatomy is tortuous and where the guide catheter does not remain in the common carotid in a stable position. In an 8 or 9F guide, a second .014- or .018-in. wire system can easily be accommodated while leaving the .035-in. wire in place.

E.   Balloon Technique

Various types of balloon angioplasty equipment are available. Peripheral balloons are mounted on large (5F) shafts and may be passed over .035-in. wires. If the nonguided approach to carotid intervention is chosen (see above), or if the diameter of the carotid is truly large enough to require a greater than 6-mm balloon, these balloons may be used. Otherwise coronary-type balloons are preferred, with their low profiles, small shafts, and lower traumatic potential. These balloons come in both noncoaxial monorail varieties and classical, over-the-wire, coaxial systems. The advantage of the monorail system is ease of use for the single-operator exchange technique, excellent angiographic resolution with the balloon in place in the guide, and low friction within the guide, while the advantage of the coaxial system is greater pushability, and ability to exchange the guidewire once the system is in place. Exchangeability is greatly increased by the monorail technique while using a protection device.

F.   Stent Choices

What strategy is then to be employed? If a stent is to be implanted, the decision must be made whether to use direct (without balloon predilatation) stenting or balloon predilatation before stenting. This decision will be influenced in part by the tightness of the stenosis to be treated and by the stability of the guiding system. If the lesion is extremely tight (<1.5 mm for a 5F delivery system and up to 2.3 mm for 7F) or if the guide catheter is somewhat less stable than desired, passage of the stent without preceding balloon inflation may be difficult or impossible. In these situations, predilatation is recommended. In either case, a "low-touch" approach should be taken, attempting to minimize arterial trauma by using as low a pressure inflation as possible consistent with opening the lesion. Once the lesion is seen fluoroscopically to "yield" to the balloon inflation, further incrementing of balloon pressure should be limited with the objective of achieving a relatively uniform balloon expansion at the nominal size of the chosen balloon.

As opposed to the coronary circulation and other peripheral beds, prolonged balloon inflations are not utilized because of the threat of transient loss of consciousness or other neurological sequelae. If balloon inflation is performed prior to stent implantation, the result must be carefully evaluated for evidence of dissection and, if present, for length and exact position of dissection, since this will have to be covered by the stent placement. It must be remembered from the outset that the goal of the carotid intervention is not the creation of a neolumen of the same size as the nominal diameter of the artery as in the case of coronary arteries. The goal is to create an acceptable lumen that has a low likelihood of restenosis and to cover the area of ulcerated plaque to render unlikely further embolic episodes. Thus the balloon size chosen must not be excessive and is usually 1–2 mm lower than that of the final stent dilation.

An argument can be made for direct stenting: less trauma without predilatation, less embolization. This has not been systematically evaluated. The downside of direct stenting is the possibility, especially in heavily calcified lesions, of a failure to dilate the lesion due to the extremely rigid concentric calcium. This may result in a deployed but poorly expanded stent that cannot be removed and will provide a nidus for thrombosis and embolization. This results in a need for urgent surgical treatment.

If direct stenting is chosen, a low-profile delivery system is desired to facilitate crossing with the least traumatic potential after which the stent is implanted either by bal-loon expansion or by the intrinsic unsheathing mechanism in the case of a self-expanding stent. Following stent im-plantation in the case of a balloon-expandable (BE) stent, the result may be evaluated with control angiography and may be sufficient without further dilatation. Following self-expanding (SE) stent implantation, postdilatation is neces-sary to adequately treat the lesion and properly appose the stent to the vessel wall. This is important not only for the immediate result, but to assure good fixation of the stent to avoid migration (36).

One of the debates that have plagued carotid stenting is the question of BE versus SE stents. Certain investiga-tors have had protocol mandates to use one or the other, but advantages and disadvantages have emerged for both systems (Table 4). What is clear is that the risk for external compression with currently available BE stents is 7–11%, and thus many practitioners have shifted to the use of SE stents (17,37). That having been said, certain anatomical situations call for the more precise placement characteris-tics of the current BE stents. The ostium of the common carotid, the distal segment of the internal, and the ostium of the internal when there is no disease extending across the bifurcation from the common carotid are sites where the precise placement of a BE stent may avoid distal dissec-tion or missing the ostium. The restenosis risk has in gen-eral been very low,and it remains to be seen whether there is a differential in restenosis with either SE or BE stents, and if so, with which particular stents. In addition, al-though it is a rare complication, migration of the stent may in theory be more likely when a SE stent is poorly apposed to the vessel wall. A particular concern must be the ques-tion of the durability of a stent placed in the carotid artery of a young and active patient. The conditions of long-term flexion and torsion stresses on stent metal fatigue are not known with certainty. It is reasonable to predict that the mesh-covered SE stents would react more favorably over

Table 4 Balloon-Expandable Versus Self-Expanding Stents

	Balloon-expandable	Self-expanding
Advantages	Accurate deployment with certainty of proximal edge Availability in shorter lengths thus allowing "spot" stenting Lower profile allowing smaller access conduits and potentially less predilatation	Minimal trauma on implantation Stent covers plaque before any barotraumas Excellent coverage of entire disease length especially in lesions that originate in CCA and extend to ICA Better resistance to external compressive force Better contouring to artery (esp. laser-cut)
Disadvantages	Potentially embologenic during implantation since barotrauma simultaneous with implantation Ill-suited to span the bifurcation, since requires differential balloon sizing for CCA/ICA Compressible with external force after implantation	Inaccuracy of proximal edge deployment May be poor choice for lesions beginning exactly at ostium of CCA or ICA Shortest length presently available is 2 cm for laser-cut nitinol stent ?Potential for migration if not well apposed Potential for flexion-torsion fatigue and breakage over long duration (laser-cut)

the long haul than multimodular laser-cut stents, which might be more prone to fatigue and potential breakage in such circumstances. At present it may be best to recommend surgical treatment in these patients.

G.   Prevention of Distal Embolization

Many of these concerns regarding the choice of tools for carotid angioplasty and stenting have to do with the most feared complication of carotid intervention, distal embolization, with its attendant parenchymal damage in the form of TIA or stroke. Reported rates of any neurological complication range as high as 6.4% (17), in Roubin's series, which was extremely strict with its reporting of these events, including contralateral strokes in patients known to have had previous cardiac embolic strokes with a substrate of mitral disease and atrial fibrillation. In a large survey of current stent use in the carotids, Wholey reported a 2.72% incidence of minor strokes, a 1.49% incidence of major strokes, and a 30-day mortality rate of 0.86%. The combined minor and major strokes and procedure-related death rate was 5.07%. Restenosis rates of carotid stenting have been 1.99% and 3.46% at 6 and 12 months, respectively. The rate of neurological events after stent placement has been 1.42% at 6–12-month follow-up (38). This is compared to the conservative reporting for endarterectomy in NASCET of 4.0% nondisabling stroke, 1.6% nonfatal, disabling stroke, and 1.2% death. Nonetheless, for the interventional technique to have a major advantage over carotid endarterectomy, the neurological complication rate must clearly and reproducibly fall below that of the surgical procedure.

There are multiple mechanisms for distal embolization (Table 6): aortic and cardiac sources as well as the carotid lesion itself may contribute to embolic morbidity and mortality. The carotid bifurcation appears more prone than most other areas of the vascular system to harbor friable atheroma with a complex structure including cholesterol

Table 5 Pros and Cons of Balloon and Filter
Protection Technique at Each Step

	Balloon	Filter
Crossing the lesion	+++	++
Stenting	+++	+++
Postdilating	+++	+++
Visualization	−	+++
Perfusion	−	++
Retrieval of debris	+++	+++
Filtration	−	+
Aspiration	+	−
Flushing	+	−
Complications of device		
Spasm	++	+
Dissection	+	++
Perforation	+	+
Withdrawal through the stent	+++	+

crystals, thrombi, and calcifications. Ohki and colleagues (39), using an explanted carotid model, found that balloon angioplasty and stenting produced embolic particles that consisted of atherosclerotic debris, organized thrombus, and calcified material. More recently, Coggia et al. found similar results in this model and showed that relatively small particles, 220 µm, were released in the early stages of the procedure, while crossing with the wire or balloon, and much larger particles, 1100 µm, during the balloon dilatation (40). The implications of this for intervention and stenting in this region are significant. Jordan and colleagues (41), using transcranial Doppler (TCD) measurements in 40 carotid stenting and 75 endarterectomy patients, found a significant number of embolic episodes during carotid angioplasty and stenting with a mean of 74.0 emboli per procedure and four neurological events in the group. In CEA procedures, there was a mean of 8.8 emboli per procedure with one neurological event in this group

Table 6 Etiology of Neurological Complications of Carotid Angioplasty and Stenting

1. Cardiovascular
   a. Bradycardia/arrhythmia
   b. Hypotension
2. Neurological
   a. Prior stroke
   b. Intracranial stenosis
   c. Aneurysm
3. Procedure-related (acute)
   a. Access/exchange
      i. Detachment of plaque (aorta, common carotid, bifurcation)
      ii. Clots, air bubbles
      iii. Dissection by guide catheter
   b. Dilatation
      i. Embolic debris from the lesion
      ii. Dissection either at the dilatation or protection site
      iii. Arterial rupture
      iv. Balloon rupture
   c. Stenting
      i. Transfer of clots or detached debris from the guide catheter to the internal carotid
   d. Postdilatation
      i. See (b) above
      ii. Squeezing of debris through stent struts (cheese-cutter effect)
   e. Protection devices
      i. See Table 5
   f. Drug therapy
      i. Intracerebral bleed (GP IIb-IIIa, clopidogrel, ASA, heparin)
      ii. Iatrogenic hypoperfusion (beta-blocker, antihypertensives)
      iii. Oversedation—loss of patient feedback to detect complications
4. Procedure-related (delayed)
   a. Stent thrombosis
   b. Compression
   c. ?Migration of stent
   d. ?Flexion-torsion fatigue and breakage of stent
   e. Restenosis

(p = .0001 for embolization). Interestingly, in the stenting group, patients who remained neurologically symptom-free had as many episodes of embolization detected by TCD as those patients who had events: with a mean embolic rate of 85.1 for the asymptomatic patients versus 59.0 for the patients who had a neurological event. Even though those patients who are classified as asymptomatic have no sensorimotor findings, it would be naive to assume that no subtle neuropsychological changes may have occurred.

Thus a number of investigators have proposed mechanisms for distal protection during carotid intervention. Theron and colleagues (42) pioneered the use of distal protection for carotid intervention in 1990 using a triple-coaxial, distal occluding balloon catheter system. The technique consists of a 2.3F microcatheter with a leading latex distal occluder balloon on which is mounted an angioplasty predilating balloon catheter. The entire assemblage is advanced across the lesion through the guide catheter, and the distal occluder balloon is inflated in the ICA past the lesion. Angioplasty is then performed, followed by stent implantation and predilatation, after which the guide catheter is advanced through the stent and used either to flush any debris toward the external carotid or to aspirate the debris. Following this, the occluder balloon is deflated and control angiography is performed. Results reported with this technique have been encouraging with a 2% embolic complication rate (43). Although this original work showed great promise, the catheter system itself had drawbacks including suboptimal steerability and radiopacity, as well as a high profile. A more recent addition to the arsenal of protection devices is the PercuSurge system, originally studied by Oesterle et al. in animals (44) and by Webb et al. in human saphenous vein grafts (45). This system is very low profile, consisting of a .014-in. nitinol hypotube guidewire with a distally mounted, highly elastic occluder balloon. The hypotube lumen is paired with a microsealed chamber device allowing inflation and deflation of the occluder balloon independent of other aspects of the system. The system is steerable and flexible enough to cross the majority of ICA lesions. A 5F aspiration catheter is provided with the system, thus allowing all portions of the angioplasty and stenting procedure to be performed under occlusion control with aspiration and deflation either after each step or at the end of the procedure depending on the tolerance of the patient. Common times of occlusion for these procedures are in the range of 3–10 min. The device is versatile, and can be applied even in previously unfavorable situations such as a tortuous, severely ulcerated internal carotid in a patient with contralateral carotid occlusion (Fig. 1).

Henry and colleagues recently reported their results with this technique (46). They were able to achieve clinical success in 98% of cases, failing to cross the lesion with the PercuSurge wire in only one case. The occlusion time (125–991 sec, mean = 503 ± 217 sec) was well tolerated in 95% of the patients. Only one neurological event was observed in the PercuSurge group of 94 lesions treated (1.1%). The CAFE (Coronary Angioplasty Free of Emboli) trial is ongoing and will address the question of the complication rate of PercuSurge-protected carotid stenting. A variant of the Theron technique has been proposed by Henry and Amor that combines the microcatheter with occluding distal balloon and the ability to move the system over a conventional angioplasty guidewire and allows aspiration or flushing toward the external carotid. Three other techniques are variants of a proximal common carotid occlusion technique that relies on flow reversal in the internal carotid to protect the intracerebral vessels from embolization. Kachel's device (47) is a 9F guide with a 3.5F dilatation catheter and an occluder balloon on the tip of the guide. The guide is inserted into the common carotid after wire passage, and the dilatation balloon is placed into the internal carotid stenosis. The angioplasty balloon is inflated as needed to treat the internal carotid stenosis. Before the angioplasty balloon is deflated, the occluder balloon is inflated, then the angioplasty balloon is deflated and withdrawn, and the ICA is aspirated by syringe through the guide. During this time, it is hoped that flow will be reversed in the ICA via collateral-als and directed retrogrades. The problem with this approach is that flow may not be reversed due to muscular arterial collaterals from the vertebral through the occipital artery into the external carotid, resulting in potential embolization upward from the ECA through the ICA despite the occluder balloon in the CCA. In addition, the published results include a complication rate of 4.3%.

Other variations on this technique have been described by Parodi (48) in which a triple-balloon system is used to occlude both the ICA and the ECA as well as the CCA during the angioplasty and stenting, as well as another variant in which only the ECA as well as the CCA are occluded during the procedure.

Finally, there are filter devices under investigation, including those developed by MedNova, Angioguard, Microvena, and Embolic Protection Inc., which offer the opportunity to trap the larger embolic debris while potentially maintaining perfusion of the ICA during stenting. These devices, which are essentially small basket filters mounted on .014-in. guidewires that can be easily torqued and passed across the stenosis, could offer the advantages of continued visualization by contrast injection during stent placement as well as the obvious perfusion advantage. Initial results from one study by the Montefiore group and Roubin's group with a filter device are encouraging, showing that the device was easily passed through the lesion and deployed, that only a small number of emboli of small size were released during passage of the filter wire, and that nearly all the larger particles were released during the angioplasty dilatation phase of the procedure. The filter was able to capture 88% of the large emboli (49). Despite this enthusiasm for protection devices, it must be remembered that these devices, especially the filters, may miss some of the smaller (<100 μm) particles, which, despite being relatively unlikely to cause major terri-

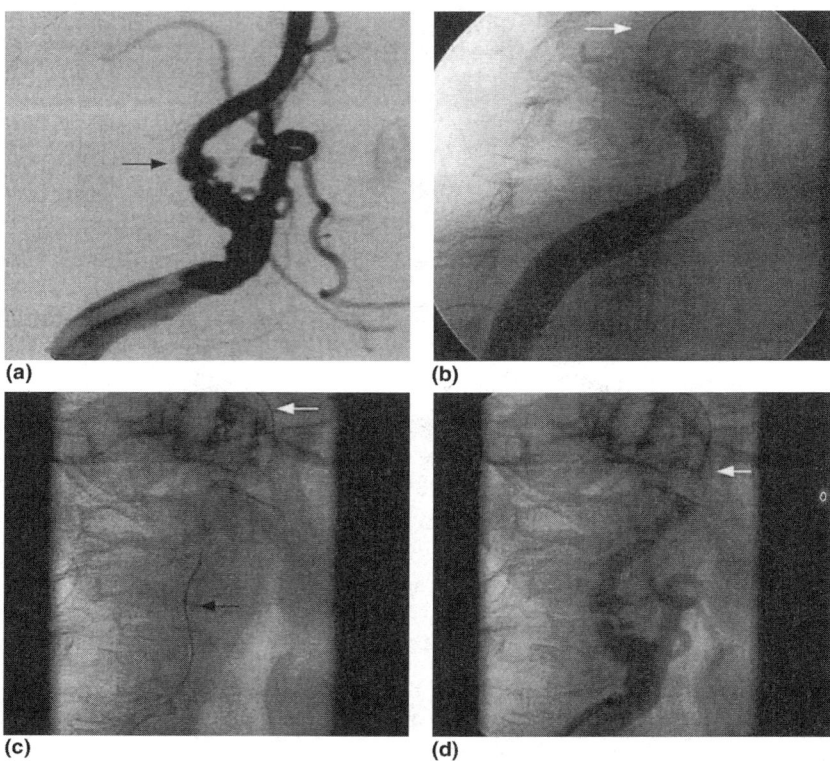

Figure 1 Protection balloon in complex internal carotid lesion at bifurcation. (a) Internal carotid preangioplasty. Note tortuosity and severe ulcerated plaque (arrow). (b) Placement of .014-in. guidewire to straighten artery after unsuccessful attempts to pass protection balloon wire. Radiopaque tip of wire (arrow). (c) With conventional wire in, protection wire is passed (white arrow) and conventional wire removed (black arrow). (d) Protection balloon inflated (arrow). Note that contrast medium fills static column up to but not past protection balloon showing efficacy of occlusion. (e) Stent implantation under protection (arrow). Visualization is maintained under protection with static column of contrast. (f) Stent after postdilatation. Aspiration catheter within

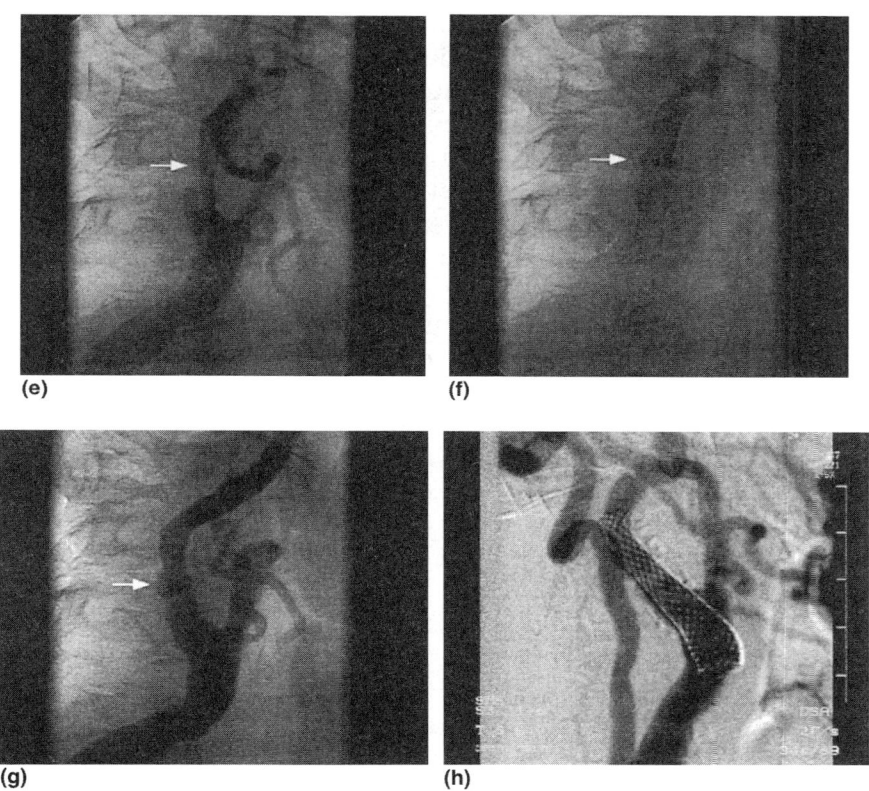

(e)   (f)

(g)   (h)

(arrow). (g) Postprocedure angiogram. Flow is returned. Note ulcers remain outside of stent (arrow). (h) Control angiogram 1 day later. Note diminution of extrinsic ulcers and excellent conformability of self-expanding braided stent to the severe curves of the artery.

tory cerebral necrosis, may nonetheless cause retinal embolization with significant temporary or permanent visual loss (Z. Chati, personal communication). In addition, there are sources of neurological insult during carotid angioplasty and stenting other than carotid plaque embolization. These include embolization of aortic debris, contrast encephalopathy, bradycardia/hypotension-induced hypoperfusion, reactive hyperemia with attendant bleeding, etc. Thus carotid angioplasty and stenting, even with protection, will never be neurologically risk free.

Finally, the question of *which* carotid lesions constitute a high embolic risk during stenting (and in their natural history) must be explored. It may well be that distal protection, if perfected, should be applied to all carotid dilatations. At present, however, protection methods have their pitfalls and may indeed induce complications during manipulation of either the devices themselves or the stent delivery systems and balloons on the devices. These complications include spasm or dissection and more rarely perforation of the distal artery. Nicolaides and colleagues have put forward a method for computerized analysis of the echodensity of plaques in the carotid artery and have examined the relationship between echolucency and the likelihood for embolism over time among a group of 96 patients with carotid stenosis, 41 with TIAs and 55 asymptomatic. All patients were examined by cerebral CT. When the likelihood of a patient having had an ipsilateral CT infarct was plotted against symptom status, severity of stenosis, and degree of echolucency, only the degree of echolucency was statistically significantly related to the likelihood of an infarct. Of plaques with an echo median gray scale value > 50, there was a 9% chance of finding an infarct while with plaques < 50%, the chance was 40% ($p < .001$, RR = 4.6). A disturbing finding in this study was that 16% of "asymptomatic" patients with carotid stenoses had had presumably silent CT infarcts (50).

The ICAROS study has been organized to assess the contribution of echo characterization of carotid plaques to the preprocedural risk assessment and lesion assessment (51).

Transcranial Doppler recordings at rest have been shown to predict further clinical events among patients with carotid stenoses, and have been used during carotid angioplasty and stenting by Jordan et al. (41) and Markus et al. (52). Mathur and colleagues (53) looked clinically at their group of patients undergoing elective carotid stenting and found, using multivariate analysis, that only advanced age and long or multiple stenoses ($p < .006$) were independent predictors of periprocedural stroke. Thus one is forced to conclude that lucent plaques and a high frequency of transcranial Doppler "hits" as well as complex lesions in older patients are predictive of cerebral events during carotid angioplasty. Were the predictive value of such an algorithm applied before the procedure sufficiently discriminative of those plaques likely to embolize, an argument could be advanced to apply cerebral protection techniques only to those lesions and patients falling into this high-risk group. Unfortunately, even the best discriminant, the computer-generated median gray scale score, could segregate groups only as well as a 9% versus a 40% risk for embolization. It remains for large studies to include preprocedure modalities that might allow the generation of a sufficiently discriminant multivariable predictive model for the risk of embolization during stenting and also for the risk of embolization from the lesion in the natural course of the disease if untreated. If validated, this model could also serve as one of the indications for stenting, since we know that percent diameter stenosis alone is at best an imperfect predictor of future morbid events in carotid disease.

VI. CONCLUSIONS

Today if one asks who should be treated by carotid angioplasty and stenting, it is impossible to answer with certainty. The earlier concept that the NASCET-excluded patient should not be considered suitable either for surgery or for angioplasty and stenting no longer applies. Exclusion today of patients who would have been NASCET-excluded for study and follow-up purposes (such as cancer) may deprive patients who might benefit from carotid surgery. It is unclear whether women will derive the same benefits as men from either carotid surgery or endovascular treatment, and future studies will therefore target the enrollment of women as much as possible. Patients whose lesions are more favorable surgically than interventionally but have NASCET exclusions that are only temporary (respiratory or other transient concomitant medical disease) should be reconsidered for endarterectomy after medical stabilization. Finally, the indications for carotid angioplasty and stenting, if it can be performed with as good or better periprocedural morbidity and mortality as surgery, especially under protection, can be expanded from those patients who are NASCET-excluded to the entire gamut of patients except

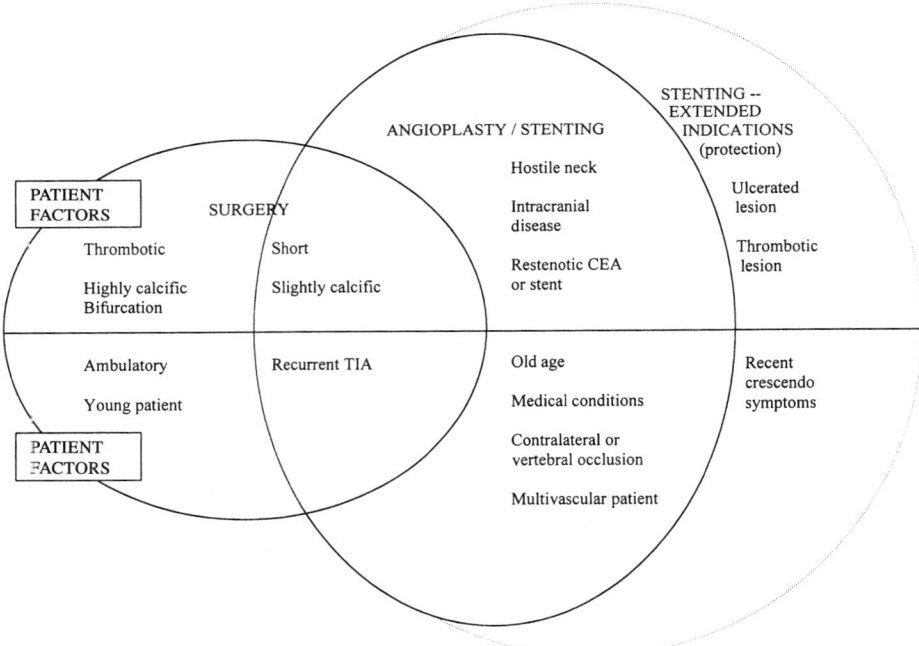

Figure 2   Current and expanding population for carotid stenting.

those for whom the lesion is better suited to surgery or those young active patients in whom the long-term fate of a stent under the conditions of flexion and torsion of the carotid cannot be predicted.

Even with the results of randomized studies in hand, uncertainty will remain since the "tools of the trade" as well as the adjunctive medications and methods of assessment are in evolution. Outside the debates over who should perform carotid intervention, and whether such interventions should be performed under protocol only, certain indications have emerged, and others will be included as protection methods are perfected and diagnostic methods and predictive models for the morbidity associated with carotid lesions come into general use (Fig. 2).

REFERENCES

1. Tan WA, Wholey MH, Jarmolowski C, Eles, G, Wholey MH. Carotid angioplasty and stenting: current benchmarks and future goals. In: Veith FH, Amor M, eds. Endovascular Therapies: Current Status of Carotid Bifurcation Angioplasty and Stenting. New York: Marcel Dekker, 2001.
2. Sacco RL, Ellenberg JH, Mohr JP, Tatemichi TK, Hier DB, Price TR, Wolf PA. Infarcts of undetermined cause: the NINCDS Stroke Data Bank. Ann Neurol 1989; 25:382–390.
3. North American Symptomatic Carotid Endarterectomy Trial Collaborators. Beneficial effects of carotid endarterectomy in symptomatic patients with high-grade carotid stenosis. N Engl J Med 1991; 325:445–453.
4. North American Symptomatic Carotid Endarterectomy Trial Collaborators. Benefit of carotid endarterectomy in patients with symptomatic moderate or severe stenosis. N Engl J Med 1998; 339:1415–1425.
5. European Carotid Surgery Trialists' Collaborative Group. MRC European Carotid Surgery Trial: interim results for symptomatic patients with severe (70–99%) or with mild (0–29%) carotid stenosis. Lancet 1991; 337:1235–1243.
6. Executive Committee for the Asymptomatic Carotid Athero-

sclerosis Study. Endarterectomy for asymptomatic carotid artery stenosis. JAMA 1995; 273:1421–1428.

7. Wennberg DE, Lucas FL, Birkmeyer JD, Bredenberg CE, Fisher ES. Variation in carotid endarterectomy mortality in the Medicare population: trial hospitals, volume and patient characteristics. JAMA 1998; 279:1278–1281.

8. CAPRIE Steering Committee. A randomized, blinded trial of clopidogrel versus aspirin in patients at risk of ischaemic events. Lancet 1996; 348:1329–1339.

9. Balotta E, Da Giau G, Saladini M, Abbruzzese E. Carotid endarterectomy in symptomatic and asymptomatic patients aged 75 years or more: perioperative mortality and stroke risk rates. Ann Vasc Surg 1999; 13:158–163.

10. O'Hara PJ, Hertzer NR, Mascha EJ, Beven EG, Krajewski LP, Sullivan TM. Carotid endarterectomy in octogenarians: early results and late outcome. J Vasc Surg 1998; 27:860–871.

11. Sundt TM Jr, Meyer FB, Piepgras DG, Fodee NC, Ebersold NJ, Marsh WR. Risk factors and operative results. In: Meyer FB, ed. Sundt's Occlusive Cerebrovascular Disease. 2nd ed. Philadelphia: WB Saunders, 1994:241–247.

12. Winslow CM, Solomon DH, Chassin MR, Kosecoff J, Merrick NJ, Brook RH. The appropriateness of carotid endarterectomy. N Engl J Med 1988; 318:721–727.

13. Bockenheimer SAM, Mathias K. Percutaneous transluminal angioplasty in arteriosclerotic internal carotid artery stenosis. Am J Neuroradiol 1983; 4:791–792.

14. Wiggli U, Gratzl O. Transluminal angioplasty of stenotic carotid arteries: case reports and protocol. Am J Neuroradiol 1983; 4:793–795.

15. Tsai FY, Matovich V, Hieschima G, Shah DC, Mehringer CM, Tiu G, Higashida R, Pribram HR. Percutaneous transluminal angioplasty of the carotid artery. Am J Neuroradiol 1986; 7:349–358.

16. Kachel R, Basche S, Heerklotz I, Frossmann K, Endler S. Percutaneous transluminal angioplasty of supra-aortic arteries, especially the internal carotid artery. Neuroradiology 1991; 33:191–194.

17. Yadav JS, Roubin GS, Iyer S, Vitek J, King P, Jordan WD, Fisher WS. Elective stenting of the extracranial carotid arteries. Circulation 1997; 95:376–381.

18. Dietrich EB, Ndiaye M, Reid DB. Stenting in the carotid artery: initial experience in 110 patients. J Endovasc Surg 1996; 3:42–62.

19. Mathias KD. Initial and long term results of carotid angioplasty and stenting: why stent? 11th Annual International Symposium on Endovascular Therapy, Miami FL, Jan 23–27, 1999.

20. Wholey MH, Wholey M, Jarmolowski CR, Eles G, Levy D, Buechtel J. Endovascular stents for carotid occlusive disease. J Endovasc Surg 1997; 4:326–338.

21. Kachel R. Results of balloon angioplasty in the carotid arteries. J Endovasc Surg 1996; 3:22–30.

22. Bergeron P, Chambran P, Bianca S, Benichou H, Massonat J. Traitement endovasculaire des artères à destinée cérébrales.

23. Sivaguru A, Venables GS, Beard JD, Gaines PA. European Carotid Angioplasty Trial. J Endovasc Surg 1996; 3:16–20.

24. Major ongoing stroke trials. Carotid and Vertebral Artery Transluminal Angioplasty Study (CAVATAS). Stroke 1999; 30:2257.

25. Brown MM. Results of the Carotid and Vertebral Artery Transluminal Angioplasty Study (Vascular Surgical Society of Great Britain and Ireland). Br J Surg 1999; 86:710–711.

26. Naylor AR, Bolia A, Abbott RJ Pye IF, Smith J, Lennard N, Lloyd AJ, London NJ, Bell PR. Randomized study of carotid angioplasty and stenting versus carotid endarterectomy: a stopped trial. J Vasc Surg. 1998; 28:326–334.

27. Alberts MJ, McCann R, Smith TP, et al. A randomized trial: carotid stenting versus endarterectomy in patients with symptomatic carotid stenosis, study designs. J Neurovasc Dis 1997; 228–234.

28. Hobson RW, Brott T, Ferguson R, Roubin G, Moore W, Kuntz R, Howard G, Ferguson J. CREST: Carotid Revascularization Endarterectomy Versus Stent Trial. Cardiovascular Surg 1997; 5:457–458.

29. Clagett GP, Barnett HJM, Easton JD. The Carotid Artery Stenting versus Endarterectomy Trial (CASET). Cardiovasc Surg 1997; 5:454–456.

30. Chastain HO II, Mt Wong P, Mathur A, Levine RL, Al-

Mubarak NA, Iyer SS, Gomez CR, Vitek JJ. Does abciximab reduce complications of cerebral vascular stenting in high risk lesions? Circulation 1997; 96:283-I.

31. Katzan II, Bazjer C, Furlan AJ, Silver M, Whitlow PI, Perl J II, Lowrie M, Yadav JS. Abciximab use in carotid artery stenting. Neurology 1999; 52:A64–A65.

32. Amor M, Henry M. Carotid angioplasty: equipment and technique. In: Carotid Angioplasty and Stenting. Nancy, France: ISCAT, 1999:139–155.

33. Mathias K, Bockenheimer S, von Reutern G, Heiss HW, Ostheim-Dzerowycz W. Catheter dilatation of arteries supplying the brain. Radiologe 1983; 23:208–214.

34. Bergeron P, Pietri PA, Chambran P, Khanoyan P, Piret V. Carotid bifurcation angioplasty and stenting. In: Veith FH, Amor M, eds. Endovascular Therapies: Current Status of Carotid Bifurcation Angioplasty and Stenting. New York: Marcel Dekker, 2001.

35. Diethrich EB. Carotid bifurcation angioplasty and stenting: the state of the art as of November 1999. In: Veith FH, Amor M, eds. Endovascular Therapies: Current Status of Carotid Bifurcation Angioplasty and Stenting. New York: Marcel Dekker, 2001.

36. Mallon LI, Endean ED. Recurrent hypertension after migration of a renal artery stent: a case report. Vasc Surg 1999; 33:329–334.

37. Mathur A, Dorros G, Iyer SS, Vitek JJ, Yadav SS, Roubin GS. Palmaz stent compression in patients following carotid artery stenting. Cathet Cardiovasc Diagn 1997; 41:137–140.

38. Wholey MH, Wholey M, Mathias K, Roubin GS, Diethrich EB, Henry M, Bailey S, Bergeron P, Dorros G, Eles G, Gaines P, Gomez CR, Gray B, Guimaraens J, Higashida R, Ho DS, Katzen B, Kambara A, Kumar V, Laborde JC, Leon M, Lim M, Londero H, Mesa J, Musacchio A, Myla S, Ramee S, Rodriguez A, Rosenfield K, Sakai N, Shawl F, Sievert H, Teitelbaum G, Theron JG, Vaclav P, Vozzi C, Yadav JS, Yoshimura SI. Current global status of carotid artery stent placement. Cathet Cardiovasc Diagn 2000; 50:160–167.

39. Ohki T, Marin ML, Lyon RT, Berdejo GL, Soundararajan K, Ohki M, Yuan JG, Faries PL, Wain RA, Sanchez LA, Suggs

WD, Veith FJ. Ex vivo human carotid artery bifurcation stenting: correlation of lesion characteristics with embolic potential. J Vasc Surg 1998; 27:463–471.

40. Coggia M, Goeau-Brissonniere O, Duval J-L, Leschi J-P, Letort M, Nagel M-D. Embolic risk of the different stages of carotid bifurcation balloon angioplasty: an experimental study. J Vasc Surg 2000; 31:550–557.

41. Jordan WD Jr, Voellinger DC, Doblar DD, Plyushcheva NP, Fisher WS, McDowell HA. Microemboli detected by transcranial Doppler monitoring in patients during carotid angioplasty versus carotid endarterectomy. Cardiovasc Surg 1999; 7:33–38.

42. Theron J, Courteoux P, Alachpar F, Bouvard G, Maiza D. New triple coaxial catheter system for carotid angioplasty with cerebral protection. Am J Neuroradiol. 1990; 11:869–874.

43. Théron JG, Payelle GG, Coskun O, Huer HF, Guimaraens L. Carotid artery stenosis: treatment with protected balloon angioplasty and stent placement. Radiology 1996; 201:627–636.

44. Oesterle SN, Baim DS, Hayase M, Ramee SR, Teirstein PS, Virmani R. A coaxial catheter system for prevention of distal embolization. J Am Coll Cardiol 1998; 31(suppl A):236A.

45. Webb JG, Carere RG, Lo K, Li C, McQueen C, Dodek A, Virmani R. An emboli containment system for saphenous vein graft angioplasty. J Am Coll Cardiol 1998; 31(suppl A):236A.

46. Henry M, Amor M, Klonaris C, Henry I, Masson I, Chati Z, Leborgne E, Hugel M. Angioplasty and stenting of the extracranial carotid arteries. Tex Heart Inst J 2000; 27:150–158.

47. Kachel R. Results of balloon angioplasty in the carotid arteries. J Endovasc Surg 1996; 3:22–30.

48. Parodi J. The new protection device. Abstract presented orally at the Global Endovascular Therapy 2000 conference.

49. Ohki T, Roubin GS, Veith FJ, Iyer SS, Brady E. Efficacy of a filter device in the prevention of embolic events during carotid angioplasty and stenting: an ex vivo analysis. J Vasc Surg 1999; 30:1034–1044.

50. Biasi GM, Sampaolo A, Mingazzini P, De Amicis F, El-Barghouty N, Nicolaides AN. Computer analysis of ultrasonic plaque echolucency in identifying high-risk carotid bifurca-

tion lesions. Eur J Vasc Endovasc Surg 1999; 17:476–479.
51. ICAROS Investigators (Biasi GM, Nicolaides AN, Mingazzini PM). Imaging carotid angioplasty and risk of stroke. Multicentre Trial Protocol 2000 (personal communication).
52. Markus HS, Clifton A, Buckenham T, Taylor R, Brown MM. Improvement in cerebral hemodynamics after carotid angioplasty. Stroke 1996; 27:612–616.
53. Mathur, A, Roubin, GS. Iyer SS, Piamsonboon C, Liu MW, Gomez CR, Yadav, JS, Chastain HD, Fox LM, Dean LS, Vitek, J. Predictors of stroke complicating carotid artery stenting. Circulation 1998; 97:1239–1245.

17
Discussion and Summary

Frank J. Veith
Montefiore Medical Center–Albert Einstein College of Medicine, New York, New York

DISCUSSION

The consensus process brought together 17 of the world's leading experts on CBAS. These 17 were asked key questions regarding the procedure and its present role in treating carotid bifurcation arteriosclerosis. All 17 expressed themselves willingly and freely.

All who participated in this consensus endeavor on CBAS felt that the effort was worthwhile. Although widely divergent opinions exist between individuals and specialties with regard to this topic, all who took part in the consensus process were surprised by the degree of consensus and near consensus that existed when the experts in the field answered specific key questions and discussed both the questions and individual answers and interpretations of these answers. Even though there were a few differences of opinion and areas of disagreement and uncertainty, these were far outweighed by the points of clear agreement (consensus) and prevailing opinion (near consensus). It was also surprising to note that differences of opinion *within* the three specialties that were represented in the consensus process were far greater than differences of opinion *between* these three specialties. The one exception to this was a tendency toward the more liberal application of CBAS by the interventional specialists than by the surgical specialists, although again there was considerable overlap between the specialties.

Even though these conference participants included enthusiastic supporters of wider adoption of CBAS, consensus was reached that clinical usage of the procedure should currently be restricted to high-risk patients. It was further agreed that widespread practice of CBAS in low-risk patients should await the results of randomized prospective clinical trials comparing CBAS to carotid endarterectomy (CEA). It was also agreed that CBAS would almost certainly have a role in clinical practice, although precise definition of that role awaits further clarification and opinions varied greatly on what that role may be. The conference participants also agreed on the importance of cerebral protection in CBAS. Because embolic particles are universally generated by the procedure, all agreed that some method to intercept these particles must be utilized. However, again precise definition of which type of cerebral protection device (distal balloon, filter, or proximal balloon catheter) will prove to be best remains to be determined.

Thus, the consensus process revealed that we are at the beginning of an exciting new treatment, CBAS. Much remains to be learned about this treatment, how it should best be performed, what stent or stents will be best, and where it will fit into the treatment of carotid disease. However, it is clear that CBAS is currently justified for certain specific indications, that it should be evaluated in other circumstances by appropriate prospective trials, and that it will continue to generate interest and controversy for some time to come. However, for the present, it is hoped that the agreement reached in the consensus process will help to guide medical practitioners throughout the world in the appropriate and cautious application of this new technology. By using the information derived from this consensus conference, physicians can apply this technology more rationally and manage their patients better in an effort to prevent strokes.

SUMMARY

Seventeen leading experts on CBAS were asked key questions regarding the procedure and its present role in treating carotid bifurcation arteriosclerosis. They also presented their data, opinions, and predictions regarding CBAS. A conference was held to discuss these views as well as the original questions asked and the participants' answers.

Based on this entire process, *agreement or consensus* was reached on 11 crucial issues relating to the current role of CBAS:

1. Widespread (standard of care) practice of CBAS should not currently take place.
2. Such widespread practice of CBAS should await the results of randomized, prospective clinical trials.
3. There are currently five acceptable indications to perform CBAS in appropriate centers.
4. There are currently five generally accepted contraindications to performing CBAS.
5. The optimal stent for use in CBAS has not been defined.
6. CBAS is not currently appropriate for low-risk patients.
7. Neurointerventional rescue skills must be available in institutions performing CBAS.
8. When cerebral protection is available, CBAS should only be performed with it.
9. When effective cerebral protection devices become available, *adequate* stents and technology currently exist for performing CBAS.
10. Assuming comparable results between CBAS and CEA, CBAS should be offered to *some* patients.
11. CBAS should *not* be offered to patients in all circumstances requiring treatment for carotid bifurcation disease.

Near consensus or prevailing opinion was reached on six other crucial issues relating to the current role of CBAS:

1. Cerebral protection devices are not currently required for CBAS to be performed in experienced centers, since these devices are not available in the United States.
2. *Optimal* techniques for performing CBAS are not currently defined.
3. Adequate stents and technology are currently available to perform CBAS.
4. CBAS is currently appropriate only for high-risk patients.

5. CBAS is not currently appropriate for high- and low-risk patients.
6. CBAS operators with complication rates equal to or better than guidelines for CEA (although the former is difficult to determine accurately) should be able to offer patients a stenting option.

Finally, there were three important areas in which there were a *wide range of differing opinions* or a real *difference of opinion* among the 17 participating experts with regard to the current role of CBAS:

1. The participants disagreed whether an FDA IDE should be required to perform CBAS or not.
2. The participants differed widely regarding the proportion of patients requiring treatment for carotid bifurcation disease who are presently *acceptable* for CBAS. Opinions ranged from <5% to approximately 100% with a mean of 44%.
3. The participants also differed widely regarding the proportion of patients requiring treatment for carotid bifurcation disease who are presently *best* treated by CBAS. Opinions ranged from <3% to approximately 100% with a mean of 34%.

Index